INFANT COLIC

INFANT COLIC

WHAT IT IS & WHAT YOU CAN DO ABOUT IT

CHRISTOPHER FARRAN

CHARLES SCRIBNER'S SONS
NEW YORK

Grateful acknowledgment is made for permission to quote from the following copyrighted material:

R. S. Illingworth, "Three Months Colic," *Archives of Diseases in Childhood*, vol. 29, p. 165, 1954. By permission of R. S. Illingworth and *Archives of Diseases in Childhood*, British Medical Association.

Jack L. Paradise, M.D., "Maternal and Other Factors in the Etiology of Infantile Colic," *Journal of the American Medical Association*, vol. 197, no. 3, page 191, July 18, 1966. By permission of Jack L. Paradise and the *Journal of the American Medical Association*.

Library of Congress Cataloging in Publication Data

Farran, Christopher
Infant colic.

Bibliography: p.
Includes index.
1. Colic. 2. Infants—Care and hygiene. I. Title.
RJ456.C7F37 1983 618.92′332 82–10473
ISBN 0–684–17779–X

1 3 5 7 9 11 13 15 17 19 F/C 20 18 16 14 12 10 8 6 4 2

Printed in the United States of America

Contents

Acknowledgments

A special measure of gratitude is due to the men and women who were interviewed at length about their experiences with colicky infants. Without exception, these parents were candid, forthcoming, and reflective. Their generosity and good humor will help others through a difficult period of parenthood.

Many people helped substantially with the medical knowledge as well as the parent perspectives reported in the book. Particular appreciation goes to Dr. Albert Collier, assistant director for health programs at the Frank Porter Graham Child Development Center at the University of North Carolina at Chapel Hill; Edward F. Brooks and William L. Beery, associate directors of the Health Services Research Center at UNC–Chapel Hill; Tony Shaddock, Ph.D., director of the New England Educational Diagnostic Centre at Armidale, Australia; attorney Hafidh Ellouse of Tunis, Tunisia; and writer S. Holly Stocking of Bloomington, Indiana.

A number of physicians contributed their time and thoughtfulness to this project: Dr. Tom Boyce, assistant professor of pediatrics at the Health Sciences Center at the University of Arizona at Tucson; Dr. Tom Murphy, pediatrician with the U.S. Air Force at Ketterling, Ohio; Dr. David Reynolds, U.S. Navy pediatrician in the

Philippines; Dr. Harold Meyer, associate executive secretary of the American Board of Pediatrics, Inc.; Dr. Lewis H. Margolis, pediatrician and research associate at the Health Services Research Center at UNC–Chapel Hill; Dr. Alan Cross, assistant professor of social medicine, and Dr. Robert Greenberg, associate professor of pediatrics at the UNC School of Medicine at Chapel Hill; Dr. James Schwankle of Siler City, and Dr. Meade Christian of Chapel Hill, both private practice pediatricians in North Carolina; Dr. Clifford David of Pittsboro, N.C., pediatrician and astute editor; Dr. Frank S. French, pediatric endocrinologist, and Dr. Martin H. Ulshen, assistant professor of pediatric gastroenterology, both of the UNC School of Medicine; Dr. John W. Denham, of the Whitaker Care Center at Forsyth Memorial Hospital, Winston Salem, N.C.; Dr. K. Patrick Ober, assistant professor of endocrinology at Bowman Gray School of Medicine, Winston Salem; at the Duke University Medical Center, Dr. Robert J. Sullivan, Jr., associate professor of community and family medicine, Dr. Stuart Handwerger, professor of pediatrics, and the late Dr. Frank R. Lecocq, associate professor of pediatrics; Dr. J. Ogawa of Seirei Hamamatsu General Hospital in Hamamatsu, Japan; and in Tokyo, Dr. Tokumitsu Shirae of Toshima Metropolitan Hospital, and Dr. K. Nishimura of St. Luke's International Hospital.

From beginning to end, unstinting time, encouragement, and advice were provided by Dr. Harvey J. Hamrick, associate professor of pediatrics at the UNC School of Medicine in Chapel Hill. In preparing the book as in so much else, it was an advantage to be married to Dale Clark Farran, researcher in child development at the Frank Porter Graham Child Development Center and clinical lecturer in special education at UNC, who provided editorial support, professional insights, and searching questions.

Foreword

We had been married nine years when our first child was born.

Married at 20, just after college graduation, I knew I wanted a career and I was not certain then that I wanted children. For eight years I worked in educational research, and during part of that time I went to school for a Ph.D. in child development.

One morning I woke up with an awareness that the time had come: I was ready to have children. (This same "sudden" awareness has occurred in the same way to friends of mine in their late twenties.) I collected the last data for my dissertation while carrying our first child, and looked forward to the peaceful days ahead when I would care for a contented infant while analyzing the data for the dissertation and studying for my last examinations. It never occurred to me that children were not something you could just tuck tidily into an already full existence.

Alice's natural-childbirth delivery was a triumph for our marriage; Chris and I worked together in a way we had never done before.

Two days after she was born, Alice began to cry in the hospital. For a newborn she had remarkable lung power. I remember sitting on the edge of the hospital bed looking down at her in amazement while she screamed. A cleaning lady in the room said to me, "What's the matter with that child?" Astounded by her question, I could only shake my head and think, "You expect *me* to know? What do *I* know about babies?"

The next day the hospital pediatrician made his standard joke about "Do you want to keep the baby?" and I burst into tears—because, in fact, I halfway *did* want the hospital to keep her. I simply didn't know what else to do.

There followed a fourteen-week nightmare. Images from that period are engraved permanently in my mind:

- My mother-in-law visiting, prepared to be very supportive because her son had had severe colic for six months. But on seeing Alice she was so shocked she couldn't help me. She said she had never seen anything like Alice's behavior. (Either her memory failed, or Alice's colic really was far different from her father's.)
- Calling a nursing mothers' support-group advisor, who told me that babies who nurse do not have colic. She said I must be "tense." I replied that if the baby would stop crying so much, I wouldn't be so tense.
- Crawling back into bed after a particularly bad crying bout with Alice and telling Chris, "There go all my dreams about being a perfect mother." He laughed about my desire to be "perfect," providing much-needed perspective.

- Reading Benjamin Spock's paragraph on infant colic over and over until I knew it by heart, and yearning for something more to read.
- Convinced that something was seriously wrong with Alice, we changed pediatricians, going to one who did what we needed most—he listened. But midway through the interview he began asking us about Alice's "temperament" and I found myself on the receiving end instead of the giving end of professional jargon. I was jolted—torn between personal and professional identities.
- Finally I developed insomnia. I was unable to sleep day or night, even when Alice was sleeping. Beginning to fall asleep, I'd have images of myself as a baby—with a big head and tiny hands and feet. The image would jerk me awake again.

After a few weeks of this routine, and finding sleeping pills only a partial relief, I returned to work. It was my own self-prescribed therapy, and it worked. At the time I was a psychologist for a social work agency. My job was to evaluate babies who were in foster care, and I could do this on a case-by-case basis. Thus it was possible for me to work two afternoons a week. I still remember the feeling of relief as the commuter train took me into Philadelphia that first day.

Working broke the spell for me. Clearly I had become too involved in Alice's colic; I couldn't quite believe that it was not going to respond to pediatric and at-home efforts. I am a classic "problem-solver," certain that any problem can be solved with the right treatment. But infant colic is one of the few problems where that approach does not work. Getting away from the situation and concentrating on something else just two afternoons a week gave me the relief I needed.

Our second child was born when Alice was five years old. He presented an entirely different case. He was a delight in the hospital and for the first week he was home. His colic started at about one and a half weeks and lasted for eight to ten weeks, occurring mostly in the evenings. When it began, I recognized all the old feelings of despair I had felt in Alice's infancy.

I do not believe the experience with the first child's colic enabled us to cope any better with the second. But Brendan's colic was somewhat easier to deal with. He had "grandmother's colic," the kind that begins when all the extra support goes home and the mother is left on her own. The belief of many parents and grandparents is that the departure of a calm caregiver brings on the colic. It is more likely that this colic is merely a late-starting variety.

The personal experience with two colicky children and the indirect experience with many more who were children of friends are what prompted the first discussions between Chris and me about this book. We knew the frustration of dealing with an acute situation about which no one had any information. If, as people told us, colic could not be "cured" and must be just waited out, at least there should be something to read. Somewhere, we felt, there should be a synthesis of what is known about the problem and what other people have tried to relieve it. And since we could not find such a synthesis, Chris decided to create it.

My personal interest in colic is also coupled with a professional investment in the developing parent-child relationship, an area about which I have researched and written for the past seven years. Several parts of this book have important connections to research and current literature concerning parent-infant relationships.

One such section is the last one where parents describe their personal experiences coping with colic. Many talk about the negative feelings they had for their colicky babies and the fears and anxieties these feelings created in them. Recently much has been written in the popular press about the importance of the early mother-child relationship. There is talk of early "bonding" and of the need for the parent to feel attached to the child. This emphasis may make infant colic even more worrisome for parents than it normally is. It is very difficult to feel affectionate toward a child who is so difficult to care for. This is particularly true of first-born children where parental expectations are less realistic and the parents' sense of confidence is lower.

Parents should know that there is very little research support for the notion that the earliest parent-child interactions are critical for the development of the child. Although the experience of infant colic is one the parent will never forget, it seldom impairs the long-term parent-child relationship. The primary reason for this is that the parent does not "blame" the child. The child grows and changes very rapidly; parents react to their children as they are at the moment, not as they were months or years ago. A strong bond will develop between parent and child as soon as the colic ends, if not before.

Another section of the book concerns family tension, specifically maternal anxiety, as a contributing cause of infant colic. (Perhaps I feel strongly about the issue because I was the victim of such an accusation with our first child.) In fact, psychologists no longer believe that parents mold the newborn entirely, being completely responsible for every trait. We are beginning to understand that certain characteristics *of the child* affect the way adults interact with it, characteristics such as "cuddliness" and activity level and, certainly, colic.

Colic could be thought of as a naturally occurring "experiment" that has been virtually ignored by social scientists. Colic is an experiment because it occurs among all kinds of babies and parents, and it is not linked to any particular characteristic of either. There is no doubt that infant colic affects the behaviors of the adults who must deal with it and that those adult reactions may in turn affect the child. However, it is also clear that once the colic is over, the effects go away as well.

My own experience leads me to believe that having a severely colicky child is like any other acute, fairly long-lasting crisis. It is terrible while it lasts, but once it is over, it is gone completely. The remnants of the experience that might remain to give the family trouble are the effects the colic had on the mother's relationship with other *adults*—such as the father, mother-in-law, or pediatrician. In this book, you will find information, from medical research to parental advice, to help you survive the crisis of having a colicky child. I hope your experience is made considerably easier by what you read here.

Dale C. Farran, Ph.D.

Introduction

A new mother sits in the doctor's waiting room ready to be called in for her four-week examination. Facing her are three other new mothers, two of whom she recognizes from her Lamaze classes before delivery. But now there is a difference.

Each of the other three has brought her newborn with her. One baby dozes in an infant seat propped on the floor at his mother's feet; another sleeps soundly in his mother's arms; the third is nursing quietly. The fourth mother feels tears well up in her eyes. "It isn't fair," she thinks, picturing the screaming, red-faced infant she left at home with her harassed husband. "Why don't we have a baby we can cuddle?"

The father of a three-week-old comes into work smiling nervously at his colleagues' jokes about his weary eyes and his unironed shirt. Finally alone at his desk, he remembers the nightmarish struggle at one A.M. with his kicking, wailing daughter. He thinks, "So this is what parenthood is all about. Why didn't somebody *warn* us?"

The mother of a two-month-old takes her sleeping bag and an alarm clock out to the family station wagon at ten P.M. She sets the alarm for one, curls up, and falls asleep almost instantly. Three hours later she drags herself out of the car, goes inside, and picks up her shrieking, twisting baby to nurse him. Then she changes his diaper, burps him while they rock in the dark, and puts him belly-down in the crib. Like a sleepwalker, she heads out to the car again.

The father of a six-week-old comes home from work at five-thirty to find his wife still in her bathrobe, hair uncombed, with the litter of baby care all over the house. Without a word she thrusts the bawling, red-faced infant into his arms and strides into the bathroom, locking the door behind her. It has been that way for nearly a month. And each evening he thinks: "We're not going to make *this* mistake again. Once is enough!"

What these unhappy people have in common is that they are all parents of colicky babies. After nine months of anticipation and the excitement of decorating the baby's room, they had a newborn who seemed fussy and fretful a week after birth, and then began crying even when he or she was full, dry, and comfortably dressed.

Then, instead of ending as they expected it to, the crying got worse—screaming and shrieking really—and it didn't stop. The agonized baby just could not be consoled or soothed or distracted.

At first the parents were puzzled, but made a deliberate effort to remain calm. Still, they watched that tiny face turn red, contorted with discomfort. The infant pumped its arms and legs, squirmed, and arched its back . . . almost as if it were trying to "get away" from something.

Their outward calm gave way to worry and concern. Was something organically wrong with the baby? The situation was so full of strange contradictions: the infant was eating well, gaining weight, and obviously strong and alert.

But the *screaming* . . . the endless, nonstop screaming. . . . Sometimes fear and anxiety were overwhelmed by anger and impatience. The parents grew weary of explaining to friends and parents-in-law why their baby was "different." At the worst moments, when their last ounce of energy and patience was gone, they even worried that they might hurt the child in an outburst of resentment. They lost sleep and resilience until all family interactions were permeated by tension and exhaustion.

Each day ended in stunned confusion: What had gone wrong?

In 1973, we turned first to a pediatrician, who told us that *our* daughter's infant colic was not injurious to her, and would go away by itself in a few weeks or months. He was right.

But that didn't stop the screaming, or the sleeplessness, or the tension and worry. We turned to the popular "baby books" written for parents . . . and found almost nothing that acknowledged the intensity of our daughter's crying and the depth of our own concern and despair.

What would have helped us? First of all, information, because to know more is to fear less. Second, advice: specific things to do to try to soothe or distract the wailing baby. Third, sympathy: the understanding of people who had been through the experience and who could tell us from their own example that it would turn out all right. We needed, in short, to feel better about our own ability to love and care for our baby, and we needed to know that the infant colic wasn't somehow "our fault."

More recently, we searched seriously for information about infant colic, and this is what we found:

- There is medical research about infant colic, and although it doesn't provide all the answers, it is more than sufficient to dispel our worst fears and anxieties about our babies and ourselves.
- Parents and many pediatricians were eager to share specific ideas for calming wailing infants and relaxing our own overstressed nerves.
- Parents who recalled vividly their own anxiety about colicky babies, their gratitude for help, and their relief and joy when the colic finally ended provided enduring sympathy and understanding.

First and foremost, this book was written for bewildered and weary parents, to transmit the information, advice, and understanding that will make infant colic easier to endure. Although a comprehensive summary of useful medical and research knowledge is included, the book is not a "Whole Earth Catalogue of Colic Remedies"; a number of "folk remedies" for infant colic have been omitted, for example, because they have never been evaluated in a systematic way.

In a sense, the book was not written for the comfort of infants at all. As our favorite North Carolina pediatrician says of infant colic, "I know the *kid* will make it. . . . It's the parents I can help the most during those eight or twelve weeks."

Unhappily, in severe cases of infant colic the parents begin to regard the child with suspicion—as unpredictable and unreliable, betraying their love and trust and expectations. We were deeply disappointed in the behavior of our colicky child, guilty about our feelings of disappointment, and even ashamed to let other people see that we had "failed" in some mysterious way as a family.

Worse yet, we found that the colicky infant undermines the parents' confidence—confidence in instinct and judgment, confidence in breast-feeding and intimacy, confidence in conscientious and thoughtful parenthood. When that confidence is gone, the ability to deal with colic and its stress is nearly paralyzed.

With your first anxious call to the pediatrician, you learn three facts about infant colic, and only one of them is comforting. First, you are reassured that while colic is uncomfortable for the baby—probably even painful—it is entirely harmless to the child's health, growth, and development. Second, you learn that colic is common—as many as 20 percent of all newborns in America have colic to some degree. The third fact is the most unsettling: infant colic has resisted all the strategies, therapies, and remedies applied to it over the years. Although it goes away by itself after a few months, there is no "cure."

Although it is common to say that the medical profession doesn't know the causes of infant colic, in fact, we do have a good idea of the *origins* of colic . . . at least some of the causes, and perhaps all of them.

We just don't know the *causes* of the causes. For example, we don't know why one child comes into the world with temporary intestinal spasms, and another does not. We don't know why one full-term newborn has an immature central nervous system, and another does not. We don't know why one child has a temporary progesterone deficiency, and another does not. But the result is the same: a bawling baby who cannot be consoled; and weary, anxious parents who need day-by-day help and reassurance.

The nature of infant colic is such that "cures" are exceptionally rare—therefore the parents' best ally in surviving infant colic is information. The information here is intended to help you get through the afternoon and evening. And tomorrow afternoon and evening. And next week . . . until your baby's system matures and the colic goes away. Meanwhile, it is assumed that you are sensible enough to seek first-hand medical advice from a physician or qualified nurse.

One mother said that in order to avoid dinner-time screaming, she and her husband kept their colicky daughter belly-down on a pillow between them on the dining room table. "All I remember about those first few months," she reported, "was that she always had spaghetti sauce in her hair."

If you have a colicky baby, that may not sound very funny.

But it will.

A few years from now, you'll have your own colic stories to tell. You'll laugh and shake your head in disbelief when you tell friends about the tactics you concocted to get through those awful weeks. It will all seem very remote, and a lot of it will seem funny.

And that, in fact, may be the most helpful information you can have.

INFANT COLIC

ONE

What Is Infant Colic?

In our family album is a photograph taken in Philadelphia in late August 1973. In the picture I am holding Alice, who was then just a month old. Her fists are clenched, her face is deep red, and her features are contorted by a piercing cry. The expression on my face says, "I cannot be held genetically responsible for this version of *Rosemary's Baby.*" My mother is standing to my left, watching. The expression on her face says, "Eight years I waited for them to give me a grandchild, and this is the best they could do?"

What is this strange condition that agonizes babies, frustrates and worries parents, baffles pediatricians, appears without a definite cause, and disappears without an identifiable "cure"?

Infant colic is not a disease—that is, it is not caused by "germs" or bacteria or infections—and it is not an organic misalignment or malfunction in the baby's body. Colic is a *symptom* of several painful but relatively minor things that can go wrong in an infant's belly in the first weeks of the baby's life.

The most striking outward indication of colic is extreme crying that can accurately be described as shrieking or screaming. The English researcher R. S. Illingworth wrote in 1954, "The screams are those of pain; they do not stop when the child is picked up; they are rhythmic, suggesting an intestinal origin; they are not due to hunger. This is the picture of the severe case of colic, and nothing can really be confused with it."

The second most striking outward characteristic of colic is that the crying baby simply cannot be consoled—at least not for more than a few minutes at a time. No amount of rocking, back-patting, carrying, or hugging will soothe the infant, relieve its pain, and end the crying. Some tricks do work, but they don't work for very long, and they don't work consistently for the same child from one day to the next.

In addition to the nonstop crying, the colicky baby typically clenches its fists and flexes or draws up its legs, arches its back, and pushes out its belly. Perhaps the greatest irony of this agonized behavior is the clear evidence that the colicky baby is an otherwise healthy and normal infant, who is active, very alert, strong and well coordinated, responsive, thriving, with good appetite, and gaining weight steadily.

How common is infant colic? Many pediatricians claim that 10 to 15 percent of all newborns they see are colicky. But research studies of infant colic commonly refer to a rate of 20 to 25 percent, and a few studies have reported an incidence even greater than that. One pediatrician pointed out that the doctor who doesn't routinely ask parents about their infant's crying patterns may find a colic rate of only 5 percent in his or her practice. But the pediatrician who asks parents about excessive crying in their babies is likely to find a colic rate of 20 percent or more.

The first signs of colic behavior tend to emerge when the newborn is five to ten days old, although colic sometimes begins while the mother and infant are still in the hospital. Colic that begins after the baby is two months old is possible, but unusual; the first symptoms at that age may not indicate colic at all, but an allergy or food intolerance.

In most cases, the colic episodes seem to cause the infant the most pain and discomfort in the late afternoon and evening, from four or five P.M. to ten P.M. or midnight. That time span is the rule, but there are a great many noisy exceptions: some colicky babies can scream at any hour of the day or night.

Most colicky infants can sustain their crying for well over an hour at a stretch, and one pediatrician reported on a group of severely colicky babies who "could cry for three or four hours without an intermission."

The colic symptoms end in some infants at six to ten weeks, but the condition has earned the name "three months' colic" because the majority of the cases seem to taper off after twelve weeks. The worst cases persist to sixteen weeks, but any symptoms that continue beyond four or five months are likely not to be colic, but food allergies or milk intolerance. Some researchers believe that colic that begins immediately after birth will last longer and be more severe, but there has been no statistical analysis to confirm this.

Many parents' anxiety about infant colic stems from a fear that their own inexperience is what makes the condition seem so intolerable. They say to themselves, in effect, "I've got to get a grip on myself; this can't possibly be as bad as I'm making it out to be."

Thirty-one parents of colicky babies were interviewed for this book, twenty-nine at great length. Although it is not a scientific sample, I am confident that this group represents the experience common to virtually all parents of colicky infants. The principal questions were: What was it like? What did you do about it?

"I remember rocking with her at one-thirty in the afternoon," an Indiana mother recalls of her daughter's four months of colic. "I hadn't gotten dressed, I hadn't had anything to eat, and we'd both be crying." The mother related that her infant daughter "screamed for four hours every day, from six to ten P.M. She screamed at other times, too, but *always* from six to ten."

A revealing story about the impact of infant colic on parents came from a woman who, on two occasions, adopted an infant right after birth. The first had been born prematurely, and had to be fed every three hours around the clock for the first three months of its life—not exactly a schedule allowing the mother adequate rest or respite. The second infant developed colic. The woman reported that the strain of providing special care for the premature baby had not deterred her from adopting another . . . but if the *colicky* baby had come first, she said she never would have risked adopting another.

All parents of colicky infants have their horror stories, but two factors seem to stand out as "unforgettable" aspects of the experience: the violence of the colicky baby's behavior, and the strain on the family produced by incessant screaming and sleepless nights.

The colicky behavior described by nearly all parents—extreme crying, "turning red in the face," pumping arms and legs, and refusing to be consoled or comforted—is not as astonishing to parents as the twisting and struggling of the infant in distress.

"It was just awful to watch," an Atlanta mother said. "She'd writhe almost out of my arms."

"Our little girl would twist and turn in pain, she was crying so hard," said another mother. "It was all so bewildering."

Parents find it hard to believe that it can take all of an adult's concentration and strength simply to hold on to a baby no more than a few weeks old. A Baltimore mother remembers that her infant son "would nurse voraciously, and then start pushing away, wrenching out of my arms."

And a Philadelphia father reports of his colicky daughter, "It was a struggle just to keep from dropping her. She'd twist and squirm and arch her back way over, and many times I was afraid she'd twist out of my grip and fall. It was like trying to hold a windmill."

If the frantic energy of the baby's discomfort is a shock to the parents, the child's sleeplessness is ultimately the severest drain on the parents' endurance.

"Our little boy could scream for three or four hours at a time," recalled one mother. "There was just no relief. And he was a very light sleeper; we had to lay him down very gently and be very quiet around the house while he was sleeping." She said, "The most frustrating time was dealing with the crying and the wakefulness in the middle of the night, because it made it so much harder to cope with everything the next day."

A woman who had two colicky children recalled that the worst one, the second, "would writhe in pain and scream from four P.M. to two A.M."

Several mothers described quite unusual sleeping patterns in their colicky babies. One said, "Listen, the 'terrible twos' and the 'fearsome fours' were nothing compared with colicky behavior." She said her infant son "was screaming and doubling up from four P.M. to midnight, and slept only thirty minutes at a time during the day. Then suddenly after four weeks he'd sleep all night, straight through, even though the colic went on for another three weeks."

Another mother, whose second and fifth children were colicky, reported that her fifth child "would flex his legs and scream from eight A.M. to eight P.M., but at night he was a good sleeper." And another recalled that her infant daughter commonly cried "from nine P.M. to three or four A.M.—and then it reversed: she'd sleep all night and cry all day." (This observation is consistent with the finding of some researchers that colic episodes can "move around the clock" in some babies.)

Because they spent more time with their infants than the fathers, the mothers interviewed were acutely aware of the stress that infant colic can place on a family and a marriage. One woman who said that her infant boy would "scream, kick, and turn red in the face" also reported, "Your family can go to pieces. With our first child my husband didn't understand why I didn't know what to do. But with our second, who was also colicky, he helped a great deal."

And one perceptive mother related that her colicky daughter "screamed and cried and stiffened her body and got blue in the face every afternoon and evening," and she reflected: "The sad part was, for five months my husband never saw her good."

Of all the large and small revelations that parents have about their own feelings and responses toward a colicky child, none is more frightening than the brief glimmer of understanding about how child abuse occurs.

"I teach courses in learning disabilities and retardation," said a woman at a large midwestern university. "But child abuse . . . now I understand it." She characterized her daughter's colic as "all-day pain" for four months. "Until she was two I was nursing the baby, I was back at work, and I was exhausted all the time. I never worried that I was capable of child abuse or anywhere near that point, but just to *understand* it is frightening enough."

The unwelcome understanding about child abuse is that it can occur not just in violent people, but among concerned, well-intentioned parents who find themselves pushed beyond their limits of endurance. A Philadelphia father, for instance, remembers carrying his colicky daughter around all afternoon in an effort to calm her shrieking, and finally, in anger and despair, throwing the infant down on a bed and saying, "The hell with you—go ahead and cry!" In retrospect, he knows he had the right idea, but much too late. He should have put the baby down to cry long before he passed the limit of his patience.

But many parents are irrationally reluctant to take the steps they know would give them some relief—and take the edge off their anxiety. The Baltimore mother explained, "If I was so frustrated that I wanted to throw the baby against the wall, how could I get a baby-sitter to tolerate it? I didn't want to impose that on a baby-sitter." The obvious answer is that a friend or baby-sitter will never reach the limit of endurance in three hours' time; but the same three hours—jogging in the park or sitting in a mild stupor in a movie theater—can go a long way toward repairing a parent's overstressed emotions and bringing the mother back from the brink of nervous exhaustion.

There are some gimmicks to take the edge off your resentment. We heard of a California woman who feared she might hurt her colicky child in an outburst of anger. Her pediatrician told her, "You really want to cuss the baby out, don't you? Well, go ahead. Use your sweetest, gentlest voice, so you don't feel guilty about communicating anger to the child. Then use all the cuss words you know—tell him exactly how you feel about what he's putting you through. Get it out of your system; you'll feel a lot better."

While they are coping with the strain of colic at home, many women have said they find themselves examining the history of their pregnancies, searching for clues that might help explain their babies' colic.

One mother remembers that her colicky daughter "was moving very fast in utero at seventeen weeks," though her pregnancy and delivery were routine. "For a month after her birth everything was easy and serene. Then *every* evening was a screaming fit." Although many mothers remember their colicky babies as being very active in the uterus, there is no research evidence that colicky infants do more punching and kicking in utero than non-colicky infants. Similarly, there is no research evidence for the commonly held belief that babies destined to develop colic are stronger or more alert in the first few hours after birth.

Three parents were convinced that the difficulty of the birth itself was a factor in their babies' colic.

"My labor stopped and started for eighteen hours," one mother said; she could never shake the feeling that "the trauma of the birth" was responsible for her infant son's colic. "He was pulled out by forceps and was in an incubator for a full day before he came to me," she said.

Another woman reported, "My husband thinks the hard birth had something to do with it." Because her child had colic episodes from five P.M. to midnight for four months, she said, "I was afraid to have more children."

A third mother said that her obstetrician decided a cesarean section was necessary, but miscalculated the due date, and the child was born at thirty-five weeks of gestation. When her son developed colic, she said, "I blamed an immature system due to the early cesarean delivery."

Obviously, since colic has no immediately apparent cause, parents cast about for some factor that may be responsible. We have a need to impose logic on this illogical experience, and so every parent *has* an explanation, even if the explanations contradict the available research evidence about colic. (For example, even after visits and calls to a pediatrician, one father looked at his colicky son's screaming behavior and decided, only partly joking, "This child was born without a stomach." The infant's mother disagreed: "He has a stomach, but he was born with only part of a brain.")

Although most colic cases end at three or three and a half months, a duration of four months is common and a duration of five months is not unusual. If, in fact, colic lasts several weeks longer than is generally reported, it may be because parents finally become convinced that they must "ride it out," and no longer turn to physicians or pediatric clinics. In other words, the final month of colic may represent a period of the condition that pediatricians and researchers rarely see. But you may be in for a nasty shock if you expect your infant's colic to disappear magically in twelve weeks because it is often called "three months' colic"; apparently the behavior frequently lasts four or five months.

What hours during the day is colic at its worst? One mother summed it up perfectly: "Whenever we wanted to eat or sleep." And it does seem that colicky infants have an uncanny ability to cut loose with their most piercing shrieks just as the rest of the family sits down to dinner. "We *never* ate a meal uninterrupted," another mother said.

Several parents reported that their infants' colic was at its worst "all the time" or "at any time," but only one—whose baby's colic lasted five months—said it was at its worst "all night." The rest were at their worst from mid-afternoon and evening to two, three, or four o'clock in the morning. The worst colicky behavior for most of them seemed to occur from six to ten P.M. The pediatric references to "evening colic" seem well founded, based on parents' accounts of the hours when colic symptoms are at their worst. Not many parents were unlucky enough to have to cope with colicky crying at two or three in the morning.

Among children described by their parents as being colicky "all day" or "all the time" (rather than limited to certain hours), it seems clear that the duration of the colic was longer—four to eight months. (As will be discussed later, colicky behavior that lasts beyond five months or so may not be "true" colic at all, but a milk allergy or food intolerance.) The "all day" variety of colic behavior leaves the mother with very little time, stamina, or mental resilience for dealing with other children or household operations. "I never even got dressed during the day," said a mother whose colicky daughter was born in New Mexico; another recalled, "I used to sit on the floor with the baby all afternoon."

Who first diagnoses infant colic, or gives that name to the extreme crying when it begins to worry the parents? Of the parents we interviewed, as many said "I diagnosed it" as "Our pediatrician told us what it was." Several said they recognized the colic symptoms from reading they had been doing during the late stages of their pregnancies; and a few said, "My husband and I figured it out." One said, "My mother knew what it was"; another said, "My grandmother told me"; and a third said, "My mother-in-law recognized it, because my husband had colic really bad when he was a baby."

So the picture that emerges from mothers' own accounts is of a condition that appears three days to two weeks after the baby's birth, occasionally while mother and infant are still in the hospital; that can last as little as six weeks or as long as six months or more, although four months seems commonest; and that is worse in the late afternoon and evening, although some families must endure it after midnight or all during the day.

Just as no one can say precisely what causes infant colic, no one can say exactly what causes it to end—although several apparently logical reasons for its beginning and end will be described in chapter 2. The colic symptoms don't end abruptly in flowers and rainbows, the way parents wish they would; the symptoms trail off gradually over a week or more . . . and often return for a few days to give everyone's nerves and endurance one last test, before disappearing for good.

Certain other kinds of behavior are *incorrectly* thought to be a part of infant colic:

- Regurgitating, or spitting up during or just after feedings, is no more common among colicky babies than among any other babies, and has no apparent connection with colic.
- Projectile vomiting (that is, vomiting with great force) is not a part of colic, though it may sometimes accompany colic; its separate causes are explained by the research reported in chapter 2.
- Neither diarrhea nor constipation are a part of colic; either condition may accompany colic, but their causes are separate from it.
- Severe rashes, eczema, or other evidence of

> allergies (such as troubled breathing) are separate from colic, and warrant a physician's attention.

Parents trying to cope with colic must overcome some old-fashioned notions about what infant colic is. Some physicians and researchers have characterized colic as "extreme fretfulness," "psychosomatic," "irritability," and "paroxysmal fussiness"; they described the child with colic symptoms as fatigued, "hypertonic" (meaning constitutionally tense), and easily startled or overstimulated.

The unpleasant aspect of most of these terms as descriptions of infant colic is that they are judgmental, rather than scientifically objective. Colicky behavior is not irritability or crankiness. It is not fussiness. It is not the behavior of a neurotic or "spoiled" baby. All these terms imply that the child could shape up if only he'd put his little mind to it. Nor do the terms reflect the violence of the infant's crying.

The difficulty of naming the condition hints at the difficulty of pinpointing its causes and finding effective remedies. In searching for clues in medical and research texts, the reader is struck by the number of dread childhood diseases that are simply no longer a part of the American parent's vocabulary: typhoid, rheumatic fever, polio, diphtheria, and so on. But while the diseases have been so dramatically controlled, the reader also notices that common health conditions—such as asthma, colic, and allergies—have remained a constant concern over the decades.

For example, in 1948 in *Archives of Pediatrics*, Donald A. Gordon traced the medical history of colic back to the French literature of 1846. He found that from 1868 to 1900 a series of German writers expressed their confusion over just what the condition was and what name should be assigned to it: arthrogryposis, tetany, cramps, myotonia, catalepsis. Finally, in 1901 a German pediatrician introduced the term "hypertonia" to describe the infant with exaggerated muscle tension and rigidity. Inadequate as it was as a complete description of infant colic, the name stuck and was used right through the 1940s. In fact the term "colic" as a common name for both the condition and the behavior is not much more than forty years old.

The same forty-year period encompasses the great bulk of research on infant colic—possibly because a groundswell of interest in the malady accompanied the "baby boom" following World War II. By itself, the research information won't end your baby's colic, but it will answer a great many of your questions about the condition and point the way toward concrete steps you can take to relieve your infant's misery . . . and your own.

TWO

What Research Tells Us About Colic

Research—highly organized and well financed—may be the single characteristic that has vaulted American medical care far above virtually all other medical care systems in the world. But the research on infant colic has one major drawback for parents: although some remedies may have alleviated colic symptoms in research studies, the remedies cannot necessarily be duplicated at home in the family's daily routine. The value to us of such research is that it is informative.

We must also keep in mind the four major limitations on research about infant colic. Let's briefly consider each limitation.

The reality of national health priorities is that there are a great many tragic afflictions that can affect newborns, and these conditions—birth defects, retardation, and so on—are far more deserving of research funds and effort than infant colic. Millions of parents would give anything in their power to have a baby with a problem as trivial as infant colic. Consequently we must keep in perspective the place of colic on the real-world scale of health conditions that need urgent attention.

A second limitation on colic research involves the incentives for research and the interests of researchers. The incentives simply are not very great for research into problems (like colic) that will go away by themselves in a few weeks; that is, the rewards are not commensurate with the effort and care that must be taken to do good research. But a researcher who makes an important contribution in the treatment of congenital heart defects, for example, can hope that there is a Nobel Prize waiting in Stockholm. The other aspect of this is the matter of personal interest. Most people who are skilled at research would find it more personally rewarding to tackle a more dramatic problem, one in which the breakthrough—if and when it comes—will yield lifesaving benefits. So not many researchers have a strong personal commitment to study infant colic.

Virtually every profession is subject to fashionable trends, and medical practice, medical education, and medical research are no exceptions. Such trends aren't necessarily bad, they're just isolated, because they are usually not integrated with yesterday's "old" theories and tomorrow's exciting "new" theory.

Medical professionals know their thinking is hampered by these trends. Perhaps colic researcher Jack L. Paradise said it best.

> *Viewed historically, theories of . . . colic appear to reflect periodic shifts in pediatric emphasis. During an era of over-riding concern with infant feeding, thinking centered on feeding technique and the components of various milks. With growing interest in hypersensitive processes, gastrointestinal allergy became implicated. The concept that the colicky infant was "constitutionally hypertonic" and destined to become an aggres-*

sive, tense adult gained currency in a period of heightened pediatric interest in psychology. Later with increasing attention to phenomena of growth and development, functional immaturity of the nervous system and the gastrointestinal tract were proposed as causes of colic. Finally, as interest turned from the infant to the parental influences which surround him, it was probably inevitable that family tension and particularly maternal tension should have become incriminated as responsible factors.

The fourth primary limitation on colic research is imposed by hasty conclusions based on unsupported assumptions and inadequate study methods. For example, in a book for parents revised as recently as 1973, the authors discuss constitutional psychology, a worn-out theory holding that "the way a person behaves stems largely from the kind of body he has." No scientific evidence is offered to explain why this should be so, but the authors go on to imply that body type predicts behavior. The endomorph, they write, whose body is "round and soft," is "typically jolly, friendly, and well-adjusted." The mesomorph, who is "muscular" and "athletic," is "constantly active" and "highly destructive." And the ectomorph (who is "thin, fragile" and "stoop-shouldered") is "likely to suffer from colic and other feeding disturbances."

Two things are wrong with this kind of theorizing. First, colic research studies (like studies in all fields) cite previous colic research studies as references. Consequently, an unproven hypothesis like the predictive value of constitutional psychology is quoted and referred to in subsequent research and never questioned or examined critically, until gradually it becomes a part of the established body of knowledge about infant colic.

The second result is that many medical students accept such material as Received Wisdom and pass it on to parents (who must bear the burden) with all the authority granted by a medical degree; eventually it is transmitted to a new generation of physicians and parents.

But the key question is: Has research helped us understand and alleviate our children's colic and our own stress?

Research traditionally begins by attempting to define the extent of the problem. That is, when we talk about colic, exactly what factors are we including?

Correlations: Where Research Begins

One of the obvious questions about infant colic is: What accompanies it? Can we identify characteristics that differentiate colicky babies from non-colicky newborns?

In statistical research, a correlation is "the tendency for certain characteristics to occur together in the same individual." Of course, a correlation may have nothing to do with a cause. Just because "A" often appears with "B" doesn't mean that one of them causes the other; nor does it mean that a third factor causes both. All we can say is that "A" and "B" appear together in a certain percentage of cases. Some correlations might have a slight predictive value—that is, where you find one condition, you can predict the existence of a condition that correlates highly with it. But that doesn't provide explanations. The search for effective ways of dealing with infant colic is badly handicapped by many untested assumptions.

Four studies, all done in the early and mid-1950s, attempted to correlate the incidence of colic with factors of pregnancy, birth, and the first weeks of life.

- William C. Taylor studied one hundred infants with colic and one hundred without colic at a private pediatric practice in Winnipeg, Canada.
- Dr. Morris A. Wessel and others studied ninety-eight infants at the Yale University School of Medicine in Connecticut.
- R. S. Illingworth compared fifty colicky newborns with fifty non-colicky babies born at the Jessop Hospital in Sheffield, England.
- Dr. Jack L. Paradise reported a study of 146 newborns in research done at the Rochester Child Health Institute in Minnesota.

Despite the fact that these studies are nearly thirty years old, no subsequent research has done as thorough a job of correlating perinatal* factors with infant colic.

None of the studies found any correlation between the incidence of colic and the mother's age, her illnesses (if any) during pregnancy, and the term of her pregnancy.

Early observers of colicky children were convinced that firstborn children and males were more likely to be colicky. But better recent studies have shown no relationship at all between colic and the sex or birth order of the child.

In reading the hospital birth records of colicky children and in interviewing the mothers of babies with colic—research that was by no means "scientific"—no correlation was uncovered between infant colic and the mother's race, blood type, weight gain during pregnancy, the style of childbirth ("natural" or other), and the use of drugs or medications during labor and delivery.

* "Perinatal" refers to all the events immediately surrounding a birth; that is, all the conditions before, during, and after delivery.

Although it is understandable for mothers to think so, there is no research evidence linking infant colic with prolonged labor, a difficult delivery, a very abrupt delivery, a premature or overdue baby, or a cesarean birth.

Only one study (of nearly fifty reviewed for this book) purported to find a correlation between colic and fetal hiccoughs. In a 1950 issue of the *Southern Medical Journal*, a Virginia pediatrician reported, "At least 50 per cent of the fetuses who had hiccoughs *in utero* had colic later, due to cow's milk sensitivity." But recent careful research has failed to confirm any such relationship—one study even found a slightly higher rate of fetal hiccoughs among non-colicky infants.

All the studies agree that the infant's birth weight has no correlation with colic, but most of them (though not all) found that colicky babies gained weight faster than non-colicky babies. In his Canadian study of one hundred colicky infants and one hundred infants without colic, Taylor reported, "By the age of three months the infants with colic had gained on the average six ounces more than the [infants without colic]. By the age of seven months the difference had increased to one pound and this was maintained up to the age of one year."

In his study in England, Illingworth found a slightly higher weight gain among colicky infants than in those without colic, but neither Wessel (studying 98 infants) nor Paradise (studying 146) found any significant difference.

Although there is a widespread belief that colicky infants are big eaters (or nursers), that is probably because they are offered an opportunity to nurse more often, either because of the parents' belief that the child is crying because it is hungry, or in the hope that nursing will calm and soothe the child. And it is true that when an infant calms down during nursing or feeding, the nourishment alone might not deserve all the credit. The sucking activity and the warm contact with a parent might also provide the comfort or distraction the baby needs.

Only one study—Jack L. Paradise's—attempted to take into consideration socioeconomic factors, but it was not a very rigorous analysis. Because of the location of his patient group, Paradise's research included an unusually high number of physicians, medical students, and nurses. He found that "the incidence of moderate and severe colic was similar among the infants of working class and non-physician middle-class families; but among physicians' infants the incidence was approximately twice as high." (Does a colicky infant come with a medical degree? Not likely.) Paradise reported, "Among the infants of mothers in the advanced education group [that is, those with nursing or college degrees] moderate or severe colic appeared almost twice as often as among those whose mothers had not continued beyond high school."

Such results can occur at least in part because the more highly educated group is far more likely to report a condition like colic to pediatricians or researchers. This may be because their education has made them more aware of research methods, or because the stresses of jobs or graduate school make them less tolerant of a screaming baby.

It is also true that more affluent or better-educated parents are likely to be more assertive with physicians, or less intimidated by a medical degree, and therefore more willing to mention their infant's colic even when the information has not been solicited by a doctor's questions. The informal surveys of hospital birth records and interviews with parents for this book indicated what most colic researchers suspect—that the condition has nothing to do with the parents' education, income, or neighborhood. One of the largest gaps in colic research is the lack of comparative studies to indicate the rate of colic among various racial, cultural, geographic, and socioeconomic groups.

Although virtually everyone agrees that pent-up and explosive gas is always a part of colic, like other correlations it is impossible to tell whether the gas causes the colic pains or the colic condition worsens the discomfort from the gas. Nevertheless, Paradise, the only researcher to have asked parents specifically about gas, found only a 10 percent difference in the incidence of excess gas from a group of infants with no colic or mild colic and a group with moderate or severe colic.

In the interviews for this book, many mothers mentioned their babies' gas; several said that their infants' burping was "very loud and hard." And most agreed with the researchers that although the baby might get some relief from passing gas, the relief was likely to be very temporary. A more complete perspective on the matter of excess gas is a part of the discussion of the structure of the infant's digestive system later in this chapter.

Researchers have also found that infant colic does not correlate with gastrointestinal symptoms. In his Canadian study of one hundred colicky infants and one hundred without colic, Taylor reported that "vomiting, diarrhea, constipation . . . were not unduly prevalent in infants with colic." Paradise found no difference—from his group of 112 with no colic or mild colic to his group of 34 with moderate or severe colic—in the amount of constipation or diarrhea, and only slightly more "spitting up" in the colicky group.

(Facts are facts, but the statistics would never have convinced Park J. White, an eminent pediatrician who was started on a long career of colic research when, he reports, "our youngest daughter, who began her 'colic' a bit early, while still in Maternity Hospital had the distinction of vomiting across the two infants next to her and into the one in the third bassinet.")

In his study of fifty colicky children and fifty without colic, Illingworth found no difference in the number of bowel movements per day from one group to the other, and a minuscule difference in the amount of vomiting between the two groups. And, he wrote, "There was no suggestion of diarrhea in any of the colic group, which is interesting in view of the often-repeated statement that all or most of the babies with colic have diarrhea."

Does breast-feeding or bottle-feeding have any relationship to the incidence of colic? Not according to these studies; the statistical differences they found could not be called significant. In Taylor's Canadian study, twenty-three of the one hundred colicky infants were entirely breast-fed; and thirty of the one hundred non-colicky children were entirely breast-fed. In Illingworth's research in England, forty-six of fifty colicky infants were breast-fed or breast-fed with "complementary" feedings; while forty of the fifty non-colicky babies were breast-fed or breast-fed with complementary feedings. In Paradise's study, 14 percent of the breast-fed babies had moderate or severe colic, while 26 percent of the formula-fed babies had moderate or severe colic.

Both Taylor and Paradise point out that the slightly lower incidence of colic among breast-fed babies may simply reflect the early change to a formula instituted among breast-fed infants who are colicky. In other words the colic rate may stay nearly the same, but the ratio of colicky breast-fed infants will seem lower because alarmed mothers quickly switch their infants to formula to try to end the screaming.

Illingworth found that the number of feedings per day —whether by breast or bottle—was the same among both colicky and non-colicky children. But Paradise found a correlation between the duration of each feeding and the amount of colicky crying. Here again it is hard to tell which is the cause and which is the effect, but Paradise wrote that the mothers' reports of prolonged feedings "were extremely useful in directing attention to errors in feeding technique, the correction of which seemed to result in a reduction of crying." That is, crying was lessened when the duration of each feeding was shortened. The question of how much, how often, and how long to feed the colicky infant will get further attention in another part of this chapter, "Manipulations and Results."

Where no particular cause can be found for a condition like colic and the correlations add up to very little, people tend to speculate even more wildly on relationships. Convulsions and breath-holding? Of his one hundred colicky infants, Taylor found three who developed febrile convulsions (that is, convulsions as a result of high or rapidly escalating fever) and one who developed breath-holding episodes.

My limited survey, however, uncovered seven "breath-holders," four of whom had colic as infants. This is a kind of breath-holding in which the baby cries so hard that its breath "catches"—its face turns blue, its back and limbs become extremely rigid, and it literally passes out in its parent's arms—a terrifying experience for any young mother or father. The baby may be unconscious for two or three seconds while its body gradually relaxes; the child usually shudders with its first breath, and then may whimper or appear very drowsy.

Pediatricians claim there is no danger in this kind of breath-holding. The parents report that it is entirely involuntary; it may occur two or three times a week, and sometimes when the child is very tired it may occur more than once a day. Then it may not happen again for more than a week. The duration of this behavior seems to be a year or two—and in each case we learned about, one of the breath-holder's parents was also a breath-holder as a child. "My mother walked me every night for colic," one mother told us. "I'd cry so hard that I'd hold my breath, turn blue in the face, and pass out. Even my grandmothers have told me how awful I was."

The relationship of colic to breath-holding is entirely speculative; it is likely that uncontrollable crying—not colic—is the connection. Of the seven breath-holders mentioned above, four were infants, of whom three had colic. The other three breath-holders are now adults (all are the parents of colicky children), but only one had colic as a child.

A correlation that *may* be significant—though no one can yet say how—lies in the high ratio of colicky children with older brothers and sisters who were also colicky as infants. Taylor found that forty-one of one hundred colicky infants had siblings also affected by colic; but only twenty-eight of the one hundred non-colicky children had siblings affected by colic. Among his fifty colicky subjects, Illingworth found eleven who had older siblings, of whom three had been colicky. Of his fifty non-colicky subjects, fifteen had older siblings, none of whom had been colicky.

Paradise found the same thing. Of his 112 infants with no colic or mild colic, 32 percent had older siblings who were colicky. But in his group with moderate or severe colic, 68 percent had older siblings who were colicky.

Only Wessel asked whether the parents of the colicky infant had exhibited colic as children: "A family history of colic was noted in 14 of the 48 'fussy' infants and in only 3 of the 'contented' infants. This would appear to be a significant relationship, but [the history] of colic in the parents of infants . . . is difficult to obtain with any reliability."

Wessel's point is correct, but one of the more interesting correlations (though it is no better than the others as a clue to colic) is the percentage of colicky children whose parents also had colic as infants. In our twenty-nine extensive interviews with mothers, we found ten of fifty-eight parents who had colic as children—about 17 percent—including one woman who reported that of her mother's six children, three had been colicky.

So there are twenty major perinatal factors that, the research tells us, have no apparent cause-and-effect relationship to infant colic. A few of them—like pent-up gas, or the number of brothers and sisters with colic—may be significant correlations, even if we can't explain exactly what their significance is.

The value of such correlations to us is that they eliminate certain factors from consideration. We can be fairly certain, for example, that breast-feeding or bottle-feeding, or the sex or birth order of the child, or the child's birth weight, has little to do with the likelihood of its being colicky. Similarly, colic is not related to anything the mother did during pregnancy or to the type or difficulty of birth.

Clearing our minds of extraneous information is a good way of preparing for more substantial questions. One such question is: How does the structure of the infant's digestive system relate to the baby's colic?

The Structure of the Infant's Digestive System

The digestive system is a remarkable piece of equipment. Its functions are so complex that it seems a small miracle that most infants' digestion operates so well right from the beginning.

The alimentary canal, where digestion takes place, consists of the esophagus, the stomach, and the small and large intestines—in a newborn, a total of about five or six feet of tubing. Before food leaves the mouth and throat it is mixed with saliva, which contains the first enzyme that changes some of the food starches into sugar.

The food passes through the esophagus, moved by wavelike contractions that carry the food to the stomach. In the stomach, the food is churned and mixed with gastric fluids containing other enzymes, which begin the digestion of protein foods such as meat, eggs, and milk. Depending on the type of food, it may remain in an infant's stomach only two or three hours.

At the lower end of the stomach the food is stopped by a ring of muscles called the pylorus, or the pyloric sphincter, until the gastric juices have completed their work. Although the food is churned and partly broken down in the stomach, only a small part of the digestive process actually takes place there.

When the food passes through the pyloric valve into the small intestine, additional digestion begins. The food is "processed" by fluids produced by the pancreas and the walls of the small intestine, and bile produced by the gall bladder and liver.

Pancreatic fluid contains three enzymes that break down the partly digested proteins into amino acids, change starches into sugars, and change fats to fatty acids and glycerin. When the food has been completely digested in the small intestine the food molecules are small enough to be absorbed into the bloodstream through the walls of the intestine. The simple sugars, fatty acids, glycerin, and amino acids are carried by blood circulation for the nourishment of the body.

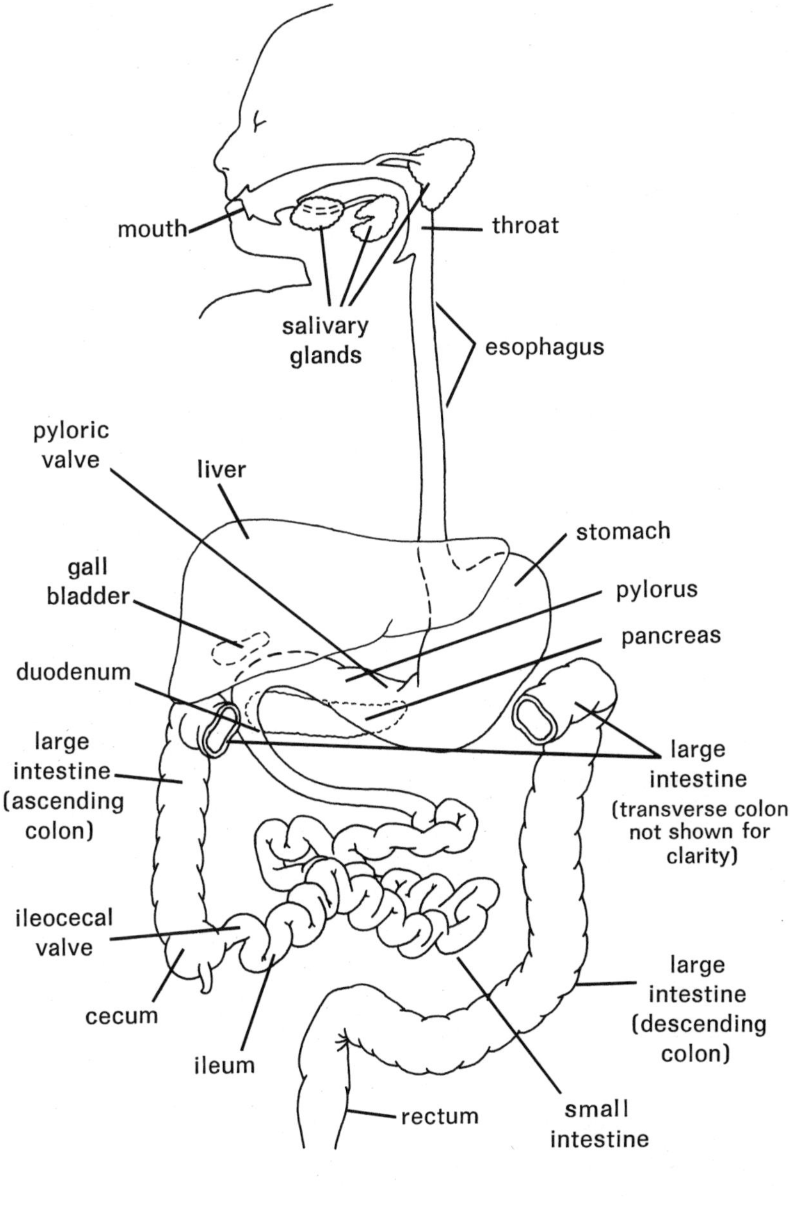

mouth
throat
salivary
glands
esophagus
pyloric
valve
liver
stomach
gall
bladder
pylorus
pancreas
duodenum
large
intestine
(ascending
colon)
large
intestine
(transverse colon
not shown for
clarity)
ileocecal
valve
cecum
ileum
large
intestine
(descending
colon)
rectum
small
intestine

The food residue moves from the ileum (the lower part of the small intestine) through the ileo-cecal valve into the cecum (the upper part of the large intestine). Except for small amounts of water and some minerals, no digestion or absorption takes place in the large intestine. The remaining food roughage is passed through the large intestine to be eliminated at the rectum.

In an effort to identify intestinal spasms as the cause of colic pain, Illingworth conducted a series of X-ray examinations of colicky children. He concluded, "The most likely explanation of the attacks lies in a localized obstruction to the passage of gas in the colon by spasm or kinking of uncertain cause."

To get the best possible picture of what was actually happening in the infants' bellies, Illingworth had X-ray examinations made of seven severely colicky children during their attacks of colic. He mixed these X rays with those of seven non-colicky children of the same age. Then he took the fourteen X rays to a radiologist who did not know the children's condition, and asked the radiologist to grade the X rays according to the amount of gas in the babies' intestines.

Illingworth acknowledged that the number of children was too small for definitive results. Nonetheless it is interesting that "five of the seven babies with colic and one [without colic] were regarded as having a normal intestinal gas content; two babies with colic and three [without colic] showed a slight increase of gas. . . . None of the colic babies but three of the [non-colic babies] showed a large amount of gas. All we can say with certainty was that in those seven babies with colic at the time of the X-ray studies there was no evidence of excess of gas in the intestine."

Illingworth concluded, "I believe that there is strong evidence that colic is not caused by underfeeding, overfeeding, errors of feeding technique, mismanagement, allergy, substances taken by the mother, or swallowing air. I do not think that it is due to an excess of wind in the intestines. I have never seen any evidence that colic is associated with . . . any particular type of baby or parent. . . . X-ray studies taken during an attack of colic did not show an excess of gas in the bowel. The most likely explanation of colic is thought to be the local obstruction to the passage of gas in the colon by local spasm or kinking."

The Illingworth study does suggest things you can do with your colicky baby. You will want to do what you can to eliminate trapped or obstructed gas as a factor. Feed the infant in an upright position, burp it carefully over a long period of time, and massage its belly gently with your fingertips to help the baby pass gas.

There is no guarantee these tactics will work well for your child . . . but they might help. And for most parents, the therapy of trying to remedy the colic can be as important to their own state of mind as it is to the infant.

Allergies: Still an Open Question

The four modern studies—Taylor, Wessel, Illingworth, and Paradise—uniformly conclude that allergies have no direct relationship to infant colic, either as a cause or as a sequel. But it may be premature to close the file completely on allergies. Because there is some information in these studies that we can use, let's review the research on colic and allergies, including a ten-year study of the two conditions.

In his study of two hundred Canadian children, Taylor gathered information on their history of eczema, skin rashes due to foods, allergic rhinitis (nasal congestion or inflammation), asthma, and reactions to innoculations. He found twenty-one of one hundred colicky infants suffering from one or more of these conditions, and fifteen of one hundred non-colicky infants—clearly not a significant difference. He wrote, "The severest allergic manifestation encountered was asthma, and this was more prevalent in the [non-colic] groups."

Likewise Wessel. Of his forty-five colicky infants, seven were reported to have a family history of "much allergy" and thirty a family history of "some allergy." Of his fifty "contented infants," seven had a family history of "much allergy" and thirty-three had a family history of "some allergy." Since the colic group numbered forty-five and the contented group numbered fifty, the difference is not very great in the percentage of allergic family histories within each group.

Illingworth wrote, "Our data give no support to the theory that the cause of colic is allergy. There was a family history of allergy in ten babies [of fifty] in the colic group and in 12 [of fifty] in the control group. One baby in the colic group developed eczema compared with four in the control group."

Paradise investigated the incidence of allergies among the parents of his 146 subjects. He found a 30 percent incidence of allergy in one or both parents in his groups of children with mild or no colic, and a 32 percent incidence of allergy in one or both parents in his groups of moderately and severely colicky children.

Paradise also investigated the existence of peptic ulcer, heartburn, or "nervous stomach" among the parents of his subjects, and found a 15 percent incidence among the parents of infants with mild or no colic, and a 15 percent incidence among the parents of infants with moderate or severe colic.

Based on these figures, the evidence seems conclusively

against allergies as a significant factor in the presence of colic. So why does the question keep coming up? Apparently because three allergic conditions—eczema, cow's-milk intolerance, and asthma and other respiratory difficulties—correlate with colic just often and persistently enough to keep parents, pediatricians, and researchers guessing.

In 1929 Dr. Park J. White, the pioneer researcher in many aspects of infant colic, reported that in forty-seven children in a private medical practice, "infants with 'true colic' in whom eczema develops later, are almost three times as numerous as infants with either condition alone." The tricky aspect of the relationship is that eczema or transient skin rashes are common enough among newborns to seem to correlate to some degree with almost anything else. Dr. Joseph H. Fries, chief of allergy at Lutheran Hospital in New York in the mid-1950s, expressed the belief (but gave no statistical evidence to support it) that "many a child with . . . eczema and severe intestinal colic loses the colic first, the eczema later, and subsequently develops an allergy to inhalants, the respiratory tract becoming the shock organ [for allergies]. Furthermore, in studies of asthmatic children, one frequently elicits a past history of severe colic in infancy."

Unfortunately, Fries did not specify the meaning of "frequently" or the specific "studies of asthmatic children" he was referring to. He did, however, institute an X-ray study to demonstrate the physical effects of food allergies in children, which showed that contractions and spasms took place in the patients' lower intestines when allergenic foods were introduced by enema.

The relevance of this research to infant colic can be questioned because the study was done on older children. Nevertheless, it is valuable to know that in severe allergic reactions to foods, "this spastic phenomenon may involve not only the small intestine, but also the colon, and even the pylorus of the stomach."

Another study related infant colic to a heavy history of family allergies. Dr. Frederick J. Martin wrote that among his patients, "a point was made of enquiring concerning hay fever, allergic asthma, [allergic nasal involvement] . . . dermatitis, frequent and severe sinusitis, and migraine headache, in the mother, father, siblings, grandfathers, uncles, aunts and first cousins" of colicky infants.

Martin apparently studied everything except the guppies in the family fishtank. To include aunts, uncles, and first cousins may artificially inflate the concept of the "allergic family." And to relate infant colic to heavy allergies in the child's parents is one thing, but to conclude that there is a significant relationship between an infant's colic and allergies in a first cousin is rather more questionable.

Nonetheless, Martin found an incidence of 36.1 percent of colic in his practice—an unusually high rate that he could not explain in his 1954 article in *Annals of Allergy*. He reported a colic rate of 60.1 percent among those he called "allergic families." Among infants from nonallergic families, 25 percent had colic—still a high rate. "Where the mother and father both suffered from major manifestations of allergy," Martin wrote, the incidence of colic was 78.2 percent. He did note, in fairness, that "a considerable number of families without allergic histories contain colicky infants. This finding coincides with our failure to abolish colic in our practice by placing colicky infants on hypo-allergic diets."

A ten-year study of allergies and colic was conducted by Dr. Frederic Speer of Kansas City, Kans., and reported in *Archives of Pediatrics* in July 1958. Speer found a higher incidence of allergy in 139 couples who had colicky babies than in the general population. For example, of the parents of his colicky infants, 7.9 percent of the fathers and 11.5 percent of the mothers had asthma, compared with a rate of 0.5 percent in the general population.

In experimenting with food substitution, Speer reported that of the 119 colicky infants started on cow's-milk formula or weaned early, 108 (or 90.8 percent) were relieved of colic symptoms by the substitution of soy milk. Of thirty-three breast-fed infants, twenty-three were relieved of colic symptoms by the elimination of certain foods in their mothers' diets: milk, eggs, corn, tomatoes, onions, potatoes, fish, legumes, chocolate, and citrus.

Speer wrote that just over 86 percent of the colicky infants who were treated by specific food elimination were relieved of their symptoms by the end of the second month of life, while in a control group allowed to outgrow colic, only 37 percent were relieved at the end of the second month.

Speer also found that among his subjects with a history of colic, 30 to 40 percent developed asthma between the ages of six and ten years. Although this connection may be problematic, the significance of Speer's research for us is that it establishes that much of what we call colic may be traced to food allergies. Identifying and eliminating allergenic foods is a painstaking process, however, and requires close consultation with a pediatrician.

The aspect of colic as a manifestation of allergy that has drawn the most attention in recent years is children's intolerance to cow's milk, and cow's milk as a possible cause of colic in breast-fed babies. Although the bulk of the research reported in this area has been done in England and Australia, a recent American study concluded that tolerance to lactose and cow's-milk protein has no significant role in infant colic.

In the *Journal of the American Medical Association* in February 1981, Dr. William M. Liebman wrote that a statistical comparison of the blood chemistry of a group of fifty-six infants with colic and an age-matched control group without colic showed no significant differences. This led Liebman to conclude that "no apparent relationship of colic with lactose consumption exists."

Liebman did, however, refer to a racial factor that complicates considerations about colic: "Lactose intolerance is an apparent genetic trait that is found in five to 15 percent of white Americans of certain extractions, e.g., European, while it is present in 60 percent to 70 percent of black Americans." The far higher incidence of lactose intolerance among blacks would suggest a far quicker readiness to withdraw cow's-milk formulas from black infants with apparent colic pains.

What is the possibility that cow's milk in a nursing mother's diet can cause colic in her breast-fed baby? A 1978 article in the English medical journal *The Lancet*, of research conducted at Malmo General Hospital in Sweden, reported: "Eighteen mothers of nineteen breastfed infants with infantile colic were put on a diet free of cow's milk protein. The colic disappeared promptly from 13. . . ." In twelve of the thirteen infants, the authors noted, the colic reappeared when the mothers again included cow's milk in their own diets.

Unfortunately, in daily life few colicky babies seem to respond to the elimination of milk from the diet. The significance of the milk-intolerance studies is that they give us something to work on. You can try eliminating milk from the formula of a bottle-fed baby, and milk and milk products from your diet if you are a nursing mother. These measures by themselves may not relieve your infant's colic—but they are an easy and sensible first step.

One mother interviewed kept a very detailed "logbook" of her colicky baby's diet, sleeping behavior, crying patterns, bowel movements, and so on. In this way she could show precise information to her pediatrician, and when she altered her own diet, she could see immediately whether any changes occurred in her infant's colicky behavior.

In fact, attempts to manipulate the possible causes of colic represent one of the larger areas of research into colicky behavior.

Manipulations and Results

The maneuvers that follow are not the kinds of tactics you are likely to develop at home as you try one idea after another. The manipulations reviewed here are fairly scientific attempts to alter the infant's food or environment in order to get a result (that is, the end of the colic) that would indicate a cause (that is, whatever was manipulated).

Some of these studies were done many years ago, before research standards became as rigorous as they are today, and others include fairly obvious biases. But the research is instructive because with an elusive condition like colic, we can't afford to ignore any potential clues. A good example is the extensive classification system of colic causes arrived at in 1957 by pediatrician Lawrence Breslow, as a result of having manipulated the most likely causes of colic in ninety bottle-fed children.

Breslow's approach was systematically to eliminate various factors in the infants' environments or diets until the colic disappeared. He started with feeding technique, personally instructing parents about the duration of feedings, the value of proper burping, the appropriate nipples for formula-fed babies, and so on. If the colic continued, his second step was to increase the volume of the feedings (to eliminate hunger as a possible cause of the baby's crying) and often to thicken the consistency of the feeding.

In those infants whose colic remained, Breslow eliminated carbohydrates from the formula. If the colic persisted, his fourth step was to eliminate at least half the butterfat content of the formula. Fifth, in order to determine whether the colic might be caused by a cow's-milk allergy, he ordered a formula free of cow's milk.

Breslow wrote, "When the symptoms disappeared with the first step and did not recur, the infant was placed in the 'feeding technique' group; and similarly, those whose symptoms cleared up with the second step fell into the 'hunger' group. If the colic cleared with any of the last three steps, an attempt was made to reproduce the symptoms with the apparently responsible agent, i.e., butterfat, carbohydrate or milk protein. Only when this could be done was the infant classified in a specific group."

Breslow found that he needed four additional categories. The infants in whom the removal of carbohydrates produced a major improvement but did not eliminate the colic completely he classified as "carbohydrate intolerance plus a second factor." There was a group of children whose colic disappeared spontaneously and could not be reproduced; Breslow labeled these cases "unclassified." An eighth group of colic cases, he found, could be made to recur based on infants' reactions to substances such as vitamins and orange juice.

Finally, Breslow was left with a fairly substantial number of colic cases that he couldn't explain. Instead of *saying* that he couldn't explain them, he classified them as psychosomatic—that is, having a mental or emotional origin. According to his 1957 article in the journal *Pediatrics*, this category was not based on any verifiable test or manipulation of variables; it was a catchall classification for those infants whose colic could not be accounted for in some other way.

Breslow gave all his colicky subjects relief from their symptoms by prescribing small doses of phenobarbital and atropine derivatives. (Phenobarbitol, though it acts as an antispasmodic, also has generalized sedative effects; it is less popular with pediatricians today as a medication for colic.) Deferring judgment for a moment on Breslow's "psychosomatic" category, his classifications are interesting.

Only two of his ninety infants (2.2 percent) responded to a change in their feeding technique. Breslow characterized the colic symptoms in these two as "severe and almost continuous," and expressed the belief that the figure might be higher among different study populations, particularly those where less emphasis is placed on feeding instruction than it is in a private practice. Ten of the ninety children (11.2 percent) were "cured" when the volume of their feedings was increased or when their formula was thickened.

Fully twenty of the infants, or 22.2 percent, had colic related to the carbohydrates in their formulas, and "the symptoms could be reproduced at will by the addition of sugars to their feeding."

The group of infants who could not tolerate butterfats in their formulas numbered ten babies (11.2 percent of the cases) and, as with carbohydrate intolerance, Breslow noted that "a relatively small amount of butterfat reproduced the colic." His figures indicate that fully one-third of all colicky children may have their colic symptoms relieved by the elimination of carbohydrates and butterfats from their diets.

The fifth group—those allergic to cow's-milk protein—included nine infants, or 10 percent of the ninety children. "All of these infants responded to the removal of milk from the diet," Breslow wrote, and all had other evidence of allergies—eczema, gastrointestinal reactions to foods later in infancy, or family histories of allergies. He referred to a 1951 report by Norman W. Clein, who studied 140 infants with cow's-milk allergies and found colic present in 29 percent. But Breslow made the astute point that "a satisfactory response to the removal of milk from the diet is [not] sufficient evidence of allergy. Neither soybean milks nor amino acid milks contain butterfat, and it is conceivable that an infant would respond well to these two milk substitutes not because he had an allergic colic [to cow's milk] but because he fell into that large group which we have labelled as 'fat intolerance.' "

The sixth of Breslow's categories consisted of eight babies whose colic was due to a carbohydrate intolerance plus some other factor. In this group—8.8 percent of the total—hunger was apparently the second factor in four of the children, butterfat intolerance was the second factor in one, and in three the second factor was never identified.

Eight infants also comprised the "unclassified" group—those whose colic symptoms disappeared and could not be made to reappear. Breslow classified an additional four cases (4.4 percent) in his "miscellaneous" group—those with reactions to certain vitamin preparations or orange juice, one with severe constipation, and one with an abnormally tight anal sphincter.

These results left Breslow with the second-largest category in his test group—nineteen infants whose colic he called "idiopathic or psychosomatic." He wrote that 21.2 percent of his subjects "failed to respond to the outlined routine and fell into the psychosomatic group." The key word in his sentence is "and"—Breslow uses it as if it establishes a *cause*, as if he were saying, "They belonged in the psychosomatic group because they failed to respond to the outlined routine."

This casual disposal of 21 percent of his cases is unfortunate, because the report was published in a respected journal and would lead an unknown number of pediatricians to tell parents, "You know, research shows that over a fifth of all colic is psychosomatic." That's the easy way out for an unquestioning physician, and it would raise disturbing questions in any parent's mind.

Breslow concludes that "the best results in the management of infantile colic have occurred when the emphasis was placed on the ingredients and administration of the formula, rather than on the emotional reactions of the parents."

With your pediatrician's guidance, you can reproduce Breslow's approach, and his systematic "one-by-one" elimination is best for identifying the infant's intolerance. Although Breslow reported that his identification system caused colic symptoms to "disappear" in some cases, other researchers are not so emphatic. Most practicing pediatricians believe that "whatever you are doing when the colic ends is what gets credit for ending it."

Make sure you are feeding and burping your baby correctly, and assure yourself that the child is feeding often enough and in adequate amounts. Get your pediatrician's advice in eliminating carbohydrates and butterfats from the baby's formula, or milk and milk products from your own diet if you are nursing. If your infant is taking a vitamin supplement, enlist the doctor's help to make sure the baby is not allergic to it. Even if this process-of-elimination approach does not relieve your infant's colic, at least you will know that the cause of the baby's discomfort is not in *what* or *how* you are feeding it.

Breslow's research was only the most recent in a series of studies that date back to 1921, in an effort to manipulate certain factors that might prove to be instrumental in causing colic. Although none of these studies has provided *the* cure that the parents of colicky children are seeking, five of them are worth reviewing.

In 1921 Dr. W. Ray Shannon published a short series of case histories in *Archives of Pediatrics* in support of his belief that "foods that the mother eats appear in the breast milk and may give rise to allergic reactions in the nursing infant." He reported, "such reactions may be in the form of skin, respiratory or gastrointestinal manifestations."

The common villain in each of Shannon's six case histories was egg or egg white; when eggs and foods containing eggs were removed from the nursing mothers' diets, colic symptoms in their breast-fed babies disappeared within a week. Tests showed the mothers or their babies reacting to other foods as well: peas, veal, cow's milk, cocoa, potatoes, wheat, chocolate, navy beans, lamb, and celery. But egg was the only consistently offending food.

Two of the six infants in Shannon's case histories were nearly too "old" for infant colic as it is normally defined—one was four and a half months and one was seven and a half months—but his theory has supporters among the nursing mothers interviewed for this book.

A physician's advice is essential in helping a mother determine whether or not to alter her own diet—and to insure that other nutritional foods can be substituted so that neither the mother nor her breast-fed baby suffers when some foods are withdrawn. The elimination of certain foods in the mother's diet should be done fairly systematically, so that if the baby's colic disappears abruptly, the parents will know which foods to avoid while the mother continues to nurse.

A different approach to the treatment of colic was described in 1937 by Dr. William Snow of New York. Snow maintained that "since infants, especially in the hospital, are kept on their backs, air that passes into the stomach . . . is trapped by the fluids usually present. Before food can get out of the stomach, it has to push the air ahead of it into the intestine."

In support of his theory that an upright or semi-inclined posture is more appropriate for colicky babies, Snow wrote, "In order to determine how often gas is present in the small intestine in the newborn . . . we roentgenographed [an X-ray process] 50 infants and found half of them with this condition. To prove that this gas had been forced down from the stomach by the recumbant posture we placed these infants in the semi-inclined position so that the esophagus would be on a higher level than the pylorus [the valve from the stomach to the small intestine] for 24 hours, and then roentgenographed them again. The gas disappeared from the small intestine in 22 of the 25 cases." In the other three, Snow said, the inclined position was not maintained.

Snow's article made clear that he was not referring to excessive amounts of gas, but to its blockage in the baby's stomach and intestines, and the child's inability to move and pass the gas normally, due partly to the baby's posture. His report continued, "The pediatrician teaches mothers and nurses to place the infant across the shoulder after feeding to get rid of the stomach bubble. We have found this to be insufficient. . . . If the baby is kept on its back between feedings, the air passes into the stomach, is trapped, and must be driven into the small intestine."

The issue is slightly different now than it was fifty years ago when Snow reported his X-ray findings; today, in the hospital or at home, infants are always placed on their stomachs, not on their backs. But what Snow called the "postural treatment" of colic is still important. One mother interviewed for this book described how she handled her colicky daughter: "We'd bring the car seat indoors and sit the baby up in that. I used to nurse her sitting up. We'd sit her up to *sleep*, even."

Snow wrote, "Placing the baby on its abdomen or right side . . . accomplished the same purpose," by preventing gas from being trapped in the intestine by food pushing through the stomach. And he added that one of the reasons that colic usually disappears at three or four months is "because the infant then begins to turn by itself and can change its position."

Of the research studies that manipulated the infant's food intake to relieve colic symptoms, none was more detailed and intriguing than those reported in 1946 and 1948 by Arthur S. Brackett in the *Yale Journal of Biology and Medicine*. Brackett's central thesis was that infant colic was a result of the mechanical aspects of digestion (that is, not the chemical ones), and colic symptoms could be controlled or eliminated by feeding smaller amounts at more frequent intervals. His 1946 article reported an attempt to alleviate the symptoms of ninety infants with pylorospasm or colic.

Pylorospasm is a temporary knotting or contraction of the pylorus, the valve at the bottom of the stomach that empties the stomach's contents into the duodenum, which is the upper part of the small intestine. The pain symptoms of colic and pylorospasm are indistinguishable in the infant; in colic, however, food is moving through the stomach and intestines at a more or less normal rate, and the infant's bowel movements are generally unaffected. In pylorospasm the contraction of the pylorus may reduce or temporarily cut off the flow of food passing from the stomach into the intestines, affecting the volume and regularity of the infant's bowel movements. (A third condition, pyloric stenosis, consists of a narrowing of the pylorus resulting in an almost complete closure between the stomach and the small intestine. Because food is then trapped in the stomach, the blockage can be dangerous, and often must be corrected by surgery.)

Brackett started with the belief that some infants have small capacities of the stomach, some have small capacities of the intestines, and some have small capacities of both. His argument was that too much food, fed too quickly for a small-capacity system to absorb, would accumulate throughout the day in the infant's stomach and small intestine. Thus the colic pains, usually most severe between four P.M. and ten P.M., resulted from the peristalsis (the contractions) of the system trying to move the incompletely digested food along. When these intense contractions occur in the stomach, Brackett claimed, the result is pylorospasm, ending in projectile vomiting. When the contractions occur in the small intestine (below the pyloric valve) the result is severe colic pain.

"Both gastric [stomach] and enteric [small intestine] colic cease in time as the stomach and the intestines increase in capacity," Brackett wrote. "Of course we cannot change the capacities of the stomach and intestines, but we can control the volume . . . of the food put into them. This can be done by increasing the number of feedings at shorter intervals [and] decreasing their size."

Brackett claimed that his theory would account for the appearance of vomiting with colic in some cases. Where both the stomach and the intestine are too small for the volume of food, "there may be gastric [stomach] colic with projectile vomiting in the early stages of digestion, followed later in the day by enteric [small intestine] colic."

Brackett's report cited a large number of case histories —of both projectile vomiting and intestinal colic—in which he had successfully "cured" the condition by manipulating the volume and frequency of the babies' feedings. In cases where he was unsuccessful, he felt that all feedings "were of a volume too large for the small-capacity stomach or intestine." Brackett warned against the rare case of pyloric stenosis: "It is well to try small concentrated feedings for a short time, but if the baby begins to lose weight," the parents must waste no time in seeing a pediatrician.

Strangely, only one mother interviewed mentioned the importance of smaller feedings, given more often—but her experience lends support to Brackett's scheme. Her first child and her sixth were "overdue" at birth. Both were bottle-fed, both ate normally, but both children were colicky and both "spit up all the time." Although she changed formulas more than once, the mother had the best result when she began to "feed very slowly, in small amounts, about every two hours." (Both children, she also said, had allergies: the first with asthma and hay fever, the sixth with asthma severe enough to warrant a three-day hospitalization as an infant.)

Another mother, whose second and fifth children were colicky, said, "I supplemented my nursing with a bottle, and overfed her; she spit up *really* badly for eighteen months. I would say to mothers, do breast-feed, but don't overfeed."

Brackett's second major article—based on cases seen in 1946 and 1947—focused entirely on colic in the small intestine, and his solution was the same—feed smaller amounts at more frequent intervals. When the valve between the small and the large intestines is too small or too tight, food accumulates in the small intestine, the contractions increase in force, and the infant has trouble.

(Any parent of a colicky child would be grateful for Brackett's appreciation of the family's "lack of sleep and nervous exhaustion." One father among his case histories, a World War II veteran, confided, "This is six times as bad as the foxholes ever were.")

Two physicians—Milton Levine and Anita Bell of New York—reported in 1950 on their experiment to find an external means of relaxing colicky infants. They started with the assumption (a fairly major assumption) that there is such a thing as a "hypertonic" child—that is, a tense, rigid baby with excessive muscle tone. This is a peculiar way of looking at a behavior without looking for its cause, but the notion had a number of adherents thirty and forty years ago. (As with correlations, there seems to be a confusion between cause and effect: does the muscle tension indicate a fussy, hard-to-satisfy baby, or does pain—back pain, headache, or intestinal pain—cause the suffering infant to hold his body tense and rigid?)

Levine and Bell wondered if helping a baby relax would cause a disappearance of its colic symptoms. They had noticed that "most infants relax completely while being nursed or when sucking their fingers," and so they asked specifically, "Could the pains of colic also be relieved by offering the baby a pacifier?"

Levine and Bell wanted to measure: (1) the success of the pacifier as a treatment; (2) whether infants sucking on pacifiers would swallow more air and thus have more colic pain; (3) whether babies given pacifiers would resort to thumb-sucking later in infancy.

In twenty-six of the twenty-eight cases the pacifier was accepted easily by the babies, and in twenty-five of the twenty-eight cases "the pacifier was successful in relieving the irritability and crying of the infant and in causing a cessation to the symptoms of colic." Of the three cases where the pacifier didn't work, two were babies who wouldn't accept it in the first place, and the third was an infant who didn't start crying until fourteen weeks of age—perhaps due to a problem other than "normal" colic.

Levine and Bell reported, "There was no evidence whatever that the pacifier infants swallowed air" in an amount that would cause them problems. Instead, "in almost all instances the symptoms of colic disappeared rapidly as soon as the pacifier was taken."

Of the children who continued using the pacifier after their colic ended (virtually all of them), eighteen had given it up at an average age of 13.8 months, when Levine and Bell wrote their report. The infants still using the pacifier apparently used it only before sleep.

Of the twenty-five pacifier users, only two resorted to thumb-sucking, and then only when they were going to sleep—clearly not an unusual number.

Given the success of the pacifier as a source of relaxation for the children, Levine and Bell felt confirmed in their belief in the "hypertonic" child: "Either the infant was unhappy because of an unfulfilled desire to suck, or the tension due to this lack of oral satisfaction causes an otherwise passive infant to become tense, which, in turn, might result in intestinal spasm and its accompanying pain."

In the parent interviews conducted for this book, several mothers agreed that a pacifier had helped their colicky babies—but the achievement seemed to be to get the screaming child calmed down enough to take the pacifier in the first place:

- One mother said her colicky baby—born a week overdue—was a screamer from 8 A.M. to 8 P.M. "I *held* the pacifier in his mouth. . . . But it did seem to help."
- Another said of her two colicky children: "Neither kid would touch a pacifier."
- And a third mother recalled: "She'd scream

> too hard to hold a pacifier. I'd dance in the living room with her on my shoulder until she stopped screaming long enough to take it."

Needless to say, the pacifier used by any child at any age must have a shield large enough and rigid enough to keep it from being worked into the child's mouth.

The pacifier adds to the list of tricks and tactics you may decide to apply to your baby's colic. That list includes Breslow's systematic "process of elimination" method of identifying problems with the infant's feeding, and Snow's "postural" treatment for freeing gas trapped in the baby's intestines by food. The list also includes Shannon's manipulations of the nursing mother's diet, and Brackett's conclusion that colicky babies must be fed smaller amounts at more frequent intervals.

Oddly enough, all the manipulations reviewed here—six major studies—gave very encouraging results. So why is colic still with us?

Perhaps research hasn't yet accounted for *all* the factors that can make a baby colicky. Also, like the rest of us, researchers tend to see what they've been trained to see. An allergist looks at a colicky baby and—presto!—finds allergies at the root of the colic. A gastroenterologist finds chemistry is the problem, but a physiologist finds the anatomy of the stomach and intestines at fault.

Family Tension as a Cause of Colic

The research reports on family tensions as a cause of infant colic range from those that are openly condescending and contemptuous of parents, to some that are merely unprofessional and thoughtless, to a few that are understanding of the problem, to three or four that can claim to be scientific research.

Let's review them in order of their offensiveness, from worst to best.

It is not exactly news that some medical and research professionals regard parents as blundering incompetents. What *is* surprising is that professional journals so readily print these judgments as if they were scientific conclusions. There are two reasons for this. One is that there are so many research and medical journals now—literally hundreds of them, publishing every month—that they have many pages to fill, and a lot of shabby material slips in. The other reason is the extraordinary pressure on researchers and physicians to publish their work in professional journals. This is how reputations are made, and the criterion is the *number* of one's publications, not their quality. And the journals themselves cannot maintain consistent editorial standards. Here's an example, from a 1961 issue of a pediatric journal:

"It is a well-known fact that the nervous mother transmits her nervous tension to her small infant in some way." This is a remarkable sentence. In addition to the "well-known fact"—no proof needed—we have the clear picture of the "small infant," which (besides being redundant) gives us an image of a defenseless, innocent baby being assailed by its mother's tension. But the author has a cure: "It may be necessary to put the infant in a hospital where the mother cannot touch him. . . . He will eat and sleep like a normal infant."

There, Mom, take *that*. Verification? Why bother? After all, it's a "well-known fact."

This excerpt, from a 1954 issue of the *American Journal of Psychiatry*, is no better. After describing a mother's attempts to quiet her crying baby, the author writes: "At this point the examiner requested the mother to busy herself with something else and took the infant, nestling him quietly. In a few seconds the crying ceased, and the infant was peacefully sucking his thumb." Obviously, Doc knows best.

Other references to family tensions as a cause of colic are less overtly insulting, but possibly more influential with physicians, because the language—though vague—is somber and restrained. But we mustn't expect these observations to be verified, either.

- A 1957 article in the *Journal of Pediatrics*: ". . . It was observed that there was marked evidence of emotional instability on the part of the parents. . . ." Observed by whom? What was so "marked" about the evidence? On what basis did the researcher measure "emotional instability"?
- A 1957 report in a Canadian journal: "Twelve of the mothers . . . appeared to be emotionally unstable" and "worried excessively about their babies." What did the author mean, "*appeared* to be"? What is the *right* amount of worrying about a baby who is crying in pain?
- A 1935 article in the *Journal of Pediatrics* states: "The temperament and emotional instability of the parents of such children often makes it possible to predict prenatally that the baby will be of this type." Proof? Verification? Don't ask. How do these authors define emotional instability? We'll never know. Did the third researcher test his theory about prenatally predicting colic from the parents' temperament? If so,

why didn't he report his test in medical or research journals?

The thing that is ultimately so disappointing about these observations is not just that they are so facile and easy to come by, but that they continue to be referred to and quoted in subsequent research articles, by medical people who should be more thoughtful, and in journals that should have higher and more consistent standards.

Some researchers, of course, have demonstrated a greater perceptiveness in their observations of parental tension.

- Dr. Morris Wessel, in a 1954 issue of *Pediatrics*: "Some physicians have described a characteristic anxious, nervous and tense parent. They have, however, not clarified whether this parental picture is the cause or result of the infant's difficulties."
- Dr. Ruth Bakwin, in a 1956 issue of *Pediatrics*: "Even the pediatrician is not consistent in his advice to the mother. . . . So, he may suggest at one visit that the mother try one thing, and at another visit something different. This, too, increases the mother's anxiety."
- Dr. Frank C. Neff, in a 1940 issue of the *Journal of the American Medical Association*: "In the narrow walls of the bedroom the crying of the infant reacts on the mother, so that she may be constantly in tears and lose sleep and appetite, all of which would undoubtedly interfere with her milk production."

Since colic doesn't have a clear chemical or organic origin, it is easy to blame "unseen causes"—such as parental anxiety. Of the research that has attempted to measure parental influences on newborns, three are notable . . . and one is not even a study of colic.

A 1967 study by J. E. Simmons and D. R. Ottinger claimed to have found "a positive relationship between human mothers' anxiety levels during gestation and their offsprings' crying activity during the first four days of life." The research was done with nineteen "upper middleclass private patients and their newborn infants . . . during pregnancy and the four postpartum days." Before delivery, the mothers were classified into a high-anxiety group and a low-anxiety group, based on their scores on part of the International Personality Assessment Test. Their babies' crying was measured by an electrical counter that recorded their crying for a half-hour before and a half-hour after each feeding. The study showed that "infants whose mothers had a high anxiety score during pregnancy cried significantly more than infants of low-anxious mothers."

The significance of the study for infant colic is difficult to assess, since colic doesn't usually begin until after four days of age. But as a study of parental anxiety and newborn behavior it is more relevant. Despite the significantly greater crying of their babies, "the more highly anxious mothers did not seem to have an immediately disturbing effect on their babies," the authors wrote. This finding seems to indicate that even under the stress of a constantly crying infant, the mothers' tension was not worsening the infants' colicky behavior.

The largest and most scientific of the studies of colic and parental tensions was the research reported in a 1966 issue of the *Journal of the American Medical Association* by pediatrician Jack L. Paradise. Paradise followed the development of colic in 23 percent of 146 infants born at a hospital in Rochester, Minn.

Paradise's bias was not hard to uncover. He felt the medical profession was not helping colicky children or their parents by its unsubstantiated insistence that parental tensions and maternal anxiety contributed to colic. In fact, he wrote, the research purporting to make that connection contained major statistical flaws and relied heavily on subjective judgments—that is, the personal impressions of the researcher or interviewer. Consequently, he wrote, "a survey of recent reviews for practitioners, and articles intended for parents finds colic attributed mainly to environmental tensions, particularly maternal anxiety."

Paradise decided not only to follow the colicky children medically, but to interview their mothers for a subjective (that is, personal) assessment of their anxiety and emotional state, and in addition to have them complete a standardized, presumably objective psychological personality test. Somewhat surprisingly, both the interview and the psychological test were given after the babies' births—the interview two or three days after delivery, and the psychological test about two weeks later—rather than before delivery.

The interviews with the mothers were designed to cover six main areas: the mother's emotional change during pregnancy; nausea during pregnancy; the mother's degree of anxiety as estimated by the researcher; her "degree of emotional warmth" as estimated by the researcher; the mother's reaction to her infant's sex; and her attitude toward her infant's crying, assessed by interview.

Paradise also questioned sources of family tension other than those stemming directly from childbirth. Problems with alcoholism, marriage, or the father's preoccupation with his career were found in the families of six of the thirty-four moderately or severely colicky children. A psychological test was given to 134 mothers; among the fifty who were rated the "most normal" and the sixteen who were rated the "least normal," the incidence of moderate and severe colic was the same. Of the twenty-eight mothers who were "cheerful nonworriers" and the four rated as the most anxious, no significant difference in the rate of colic was found.

The test claimed to measure "varying degrees of inclination toward patterns of masculine interest," whatever that means. The rate of moderate and severe colic among the infants of the more "masculine" mothers was lower than the rate among those of the more "feminine" mothers. Additionally, the incidence of moderate and severe colic was the same among the mothers the test rated as "energetic and enthusiastic," and among those who were rated "apathetic" and less energetic.

One of the results that intrigued Paradise was the "lack of consistent correlation between the [anxiety score on the test] and the author's [personal] assessment of the mothers' anxiety. Thus of the ten mothers considered [by the author's judgment] to manifest marked anxiety, only one had an elevated [test] score; conversely, of the six mothers with elevated [test] scores, only one had been considered moderately anxious [in the personal interview]." This observation is an important commentary on the validity of so much research on family tensions and infant colic, which relies heavily on the personal judgments of the researchers.

Ultimately, Paradise concluded that "no maternal factor or combination of factors was found associated with colic with any degree of consistency." He acknowledged that "colic occurred very infrequently among infants whose mothers were free of both depression and heightened emotional tension during their pregnancies." But on balance, he wrote, three findings suggest that maternal emotional factors do not play a major role in the development of colic: (1) "most mothers of infants with colic were emotionally 'normal' both as estimated clinically and as measured by the [psychological test]"; (2) the rate of colic "was strikingly uniform among infants whose mothers expressed divergent attitudes and feeling tones about their infants, and were of contrasting personality types"; (3) the incidence of colic in Paradise's own study was highly similar to those in four other major studies [Illingworth, Wessel, Brazelton, and Taylor] "despite appreciable dissimilarities among the various study populations."

(As he followed the 146 infants, Paradise found 112 with no colic or only mild fussing, and 34 with colic that was moderate or severe. He recorded that in attempting to treat the colic of the moderate and severe cases, 11 of 14 found "complete but temporary respite" during rides in a car—a form of "therapy" that many mothers have mentioned, but that becomes increasingly impractical and expensive. He found limited improvement in some infants by increasing their food intake, or with the use of a sedative drug or pacifier. But changes in the formulas of bottle-fed infants proved to be ineffective.)

Paradise correctly understood some of the reasons why "widespread professional support" should persist for the maternal-anxiety theory: "Maternal emotional factors undoubtedly do influence . . . the impressions about colic which physicians gain from clinical experience: aggressive or anxious mothers—especially if they are articulate—are the ones most likely to bring colic to the physician's attention and to register on his memory." But this is quite different from the evidence, he wrote, which "does not support the frequently stated view that colic results from an unfavorable emotional climate created by an inexperienced, anxious, hostile or un-motherly mother. By so advising parents, physicians may relieve them of unwarranted self-blame and anxiety."

But the Great Guilt Trip is still remarkably in vogue. Another researcher, barely two years after Paradise's report, returned to the notion of maternal anxiety with a slightly different angle. Situational stresses, he wrote—the circumstances surrounding pregnancy, childbirth, family support, and interactions—may be more closely tied to the development of infant colic than maternal personality factors. And the interviews for this book indicate that many parents agree with his idea—not as a cause of colic, but as a contributor to its perceived severity.

In a 1968 issue of *Clinical Pediatrics*, William B. Carey of Pennsylvania described his two-year research with 103 newborn infants and their mothers. Most of the families were middle class; all were white; and 50 of the 103 were firstborn children. Carey had identified what he felt were two important flaws in Paradise's study.

First, said Carey, "Paradise's own interview data are contrary to his conclusions. The mothers who reported being tense, depressed or both during pregnancy had significantly more moderately or severely colicky babies." Second, he wrote, the particular psychological test that Paradise used "is designed to find only abnormal personality traits. It does not measure the important situational stresses, such as a difficult pregnancy or friction with relatives."

Carey may have been right on both counts. Paradise had acknowledged the higher rate of colic among mothers who reported more emotional pregnancies. But he had also characterized his psychological test—wrongly—as a reliable measure of "normal" personality traits. Carey's definition of the test is more accurate—but it might still have been the best test for Paradise to use. Paradise's stated purpose was to find out whether the mothers of colicky children had any abnormal or unusual personality characteristics (in terms of hostility, tension, anxiety, pessimism, etc.). The test he chose should have revealed such traits if they existed, even though he defined the test's purpose incorrectly in his 1966 report.

Carey set about developing a thirty-minute interview, which he conducted with mothers within a few days after the delivery of their babies "to rate the extent and nature of any maternal anxiety." Depending, of course, on the integrity of the researcher and the candor of the subject, interviews can accurately reveal an individual's feelings at a given point.

Each mother was questioned about six specific areas of her own perceptions: the quality of her childhood experience and her relationship to her own mother; her previous experience in bearing and raising children: her emotional reaction to the pregnancy itself; her feelings about expected family supports at home; other life situations of the family, physical, psychological, and social; and her attitude toward the infant.

Carey established a scoring system to rate the mothers' anxiety as reported during the interviews; thus he characterized 40 of the 103 mothers as anxious. Of the 103 infants, 13 developed colic. Eight were girls and 5 were boys; none had any apparent food allergies. Only 2 (3.2 percent) were from the group of 63 mothers who had expressed no anxiety; 11 colicky children (27.5 percent) were from the group of 40 women who had expressed anxiety. The difference, according to Carey, was "highly significant" statistically.

Among the anxious mothers who had colicky babies, the sources of their anxiety were (in order): concern over the outcome of the pregnancy; their own experience as children; anxiety about family supports at home; other life situations, such as social or stressful conditions within the family; their experience with other children; and their attitude toward the newborn.

Carey noted that "a variety of anxieties, whether as a result of the mother's personality or due to current situational stresses, may make it difficult for the mother to respond appropriately to the infant's needs." In addition, he pointed out that "since three out of five mothers expecting trouble in their family supports had colicky babies, this form of anxiety appears to have the greatest predictive value." And, of course, if that particular apprehension is justified by subsequent events at home, the perception of the colic and the task of coping with it will be far more difficult.

He acknowledged, "Most mothers who revealed anxiety did not have fussy babies." And two of the thirteen colicky babies did not have mothers who appeared unduly anxious before, during, or even after the colic developed.

For treatment of the colicky children, Carey recommended "a quiet environment, a minimum of unnecessary handling, and correction of any faulty feeding technique." In truth, this must be said to be a fairly simplistic and unrealistic approach to the far more complex and persistent problem Carey describes. He used sedatives and an antispasmodic drug in the severe cases; and he urged the use of a pacifier. Ten of the thirteen colicky babies "improved greatly" or ended their colic completely within a few days of starting this therapy, Carey claimed.

The significance of Carey's research lies in his statistical correlation of anxious mothers and colicky children, and his separation of "situational stresses" from personality factors. The mothers I interviewed provided specific examples of how these stresses can occur.

- The North Carolina mother whose second and fifth children were colicky said, "My first child was born in 1965, and in 1966 I had a baby stillborn. Then the one born in 1967 was colicky. So I sort of blamed the colic on my apprehension, because of the stillbirth of the previous baby."
- Another mother had four children, all colicky to some degree. Her fourth, by far the easiest, was born at home ("comfortably, no lights, no shots, in the same bed") . . . a correlation that probably means absolutely nothing. But situational stresses? With the birth of her third, she said, "I had three kids under three years of age, immediately had gall-bladder surgery, and then we moved to a new town."
- And a mother whose daughter's colic was severe enough to have her described as "our first and only child" reported, "We saw a doctor—a resident at the hospital—who made me feel it was my tension, my anxiety. I got to the point where I didn't want to call her."

In 1974 Benjamin A. Shaver reported research on maternal personality and adaptation to infant colic—with results in direct contradiction to Carey's findings. Shaver wrote, "If colic were due primarily to the mother's mood and level of anxiety, we would expect the symptom to begin in the first few days of life when the mother is the most anxious and unsure of herself, rather than later when she is more accustomed to mothering. Also, we would expect the first-born of several children to be the most colic prone. This is not the case, however, for ordinal position within the family does not appear to be correlated with development of colic."

Shaver studied fifty-seven mothers from the second trimester of pregnancy through the first six postpartum months. Twelve of them (21 percent) had colicky infants. Shaver used a long list of personality measures to compare the mothers of the colicky infants with the mothers of the non-colicky infants.

"The mothers of the colicky infants were no less sensitive and responsive" to their babies' needs, Shaver found. "The mother's psychological adaptation to the infant was not statistically different when the colic and non-colic groups were compared. The reaction of the colic mother to the dependency of her infant and his physical needs was the same as that of her non-colic counterpart, and she was no more anxious regarding her overall adequacy as a mother."

Shaver noted that the "current personality" of mothers in the two groups was comparable. "Both groups of mothers had been equally successful in achieving an adult role, and both displayed a comparable capacity for closeness and ability to accept help when offered." Also, he wrote, "Stresses were comparable for both groups during the study period."

He found that, understandably, "at the twelve-week rating period, the mother of the colicky infant was definitely less confident in coping with her infant. By the time the infant was twenty-four weeks old, two months after colic ceased to be a problem, the mother's confidence had returned and there appeared to be no significant difference between the two groups."

He concluded: "We have found no statistical differences in current personality, current stresses, and maternal adaptation" between the mothers of colicky and non-colicky infants. This suggests, he wrote, "that the mother's personality, anxiety level, and degree of success in adapting to the maternal role were not factors in the development of colic in the infants studied."

Shaver acknowledged that "it is quite apparent from the data . . . that infantile colic does have an appreciable impact on the mother. Women almost uniformly respond to a colicky infant with a sense of frustration and futility."

A related issue that requires further investigation is the extremely low reported rate of infant colic in institutions —hospitals, orphanages, special facilities for newborns. For years physicians and researchers used this fact to substantiate a belief that colic is the result of a faulty interaction between parents and child. A 1950 report by Dr. Harris Levin of Philadelphia outlined the question, which research still hasn't answered satisfactorily: Is colic not found in institutions because it doesn't exist there, or because institutional staffs are too undermanned and overworked to notice and report a baby who merely cries a great deal?

In the mid-1940s Dr. Levin worked in the pediatric service of the New York Foundling Hospital. His colic study included all babies under six months of age admitted there from January 1944 to December 1947. The total of 844 babies included 645 under three months of age and 199 from three months to six months old. The duration of stay varied from a few days to over a year; the average length of stay was four to five months, both for the entire group and for the infants under three months old.

Among the 844 babies, over a period of four years, "not one diagnosis of infantile colic was made by the members of the medical staff," Levin wrote. In going back over the hospital's records, however, eight "typical cases" of colic were found—a rate of 1.25 percent among those under three months of age, and just 0.95 percent for the group as a whole.

Of the eight colic cases, the average age at the onset of colic symptoms was forty-two days—making them unusually "old" for the onset of colic. Another strange feature of these cases is that although two of the colicky infants had an adequate weight gain, the other six had a poor weight gain or a loss of weight—virtually the only report in the entire range of colic research of weight gains being less than normal.

The duration of the colic symptoms in the eight infants averaged twenty days. Two of the infants received no treatment; the other six had phenobarbital, enemas, and dietary changes.

Levin theorized that the low rate of colic in institutions could be attributed to: (1) the failure of nurses to note the condition or call physicians' attention to it; (2) the failure of physicians to diagnose it correctly; or (3) some other unknown factor. He wrote, "Since almost all wards for infants suffer from a . . . dearth of nursing personnel and since the 'normal' amount of crying is so great, it is obvious that some crying, normal or abnormal, will go unnoticed or unheeded by the nurses." Also, Levin noted, "Nurses whose experiences have been confined solely to institutions have seen little or no colic and are not 'colic conscious.' Consequently, these nurses may not note or recognize the symptoms of colic and may erroneously report or record them as 'hunger, irritability, fretfulness,' etc."

Levin believed that some "emotional" factor in the infants was also a part of the low rate of colic in institutions, but he could not suggest what it might be. Many physicians today believe it is simply a matter of reporting:

overworked nursery staffs cannot pay much attention to a baby that is well and gaining weight adequately, no matter how much it cries.

The Unknown Factors: Body Chemistry and the Nervous System

Logic—but little research evidence—points to three additional likely causes of infant colic: inadequate enzyme production in the newborn's stomach; a tardy production of the hormone progesterone in some infants; and an immature central nervous system. Let's examine how these conditions seem to be related to infant colic.

In infants an enzyme called lipase digests fat in the stomach, and an enzyme called lactase breaks down lactose, which is a type of sugar in milk. If these enzymes are not present in sufficient quantity in the infant's system, butterfats and carbohydrates in milk will be harder to digest. Very little research has been done on enzyme production and efficiency in newborns, and the proportion of colic that may be attributable to a temporary enzyme deficiency cannot be judged until additional studies add to our knowledge about digestion in infants.

The effects of hormones on newborns' digestive systems were addressed in a study of the body's production of progesterone, a hormone that affects smooth-muscle activity. It is manufactured principally within the adrenal gland system, and may stimulate the relaxation of some internal muscles. In fact, the relationship of progesterone to colic was suggested to Dr. William L. Bradford at the University of Rochester in the early 1960s when he recalled that the withdrawal of progesterone from a mother prior to childbirth leads to intense contraction of the uterus and the expulsion of the fetus.

This observation led to a 1963 report in *Pediatrics* by Bradford and other researchers in pediatrics and endocrinology (the study of glands and hormones). The authors wrote that "in certain instances the occurrence of colic symptoms may correlate with a deficiency" of the hormone progesterone.

It is known that newborns have a residue of progesterone in their bodies, which they accumulated from the placenta of the mother prior to birth. But this residual progesterone passes out of their bodies in urine as a chemical called pregnanediol. Then it may be several days or several weeks before the infant's own adrenal glands begin to manufacture progesterone.

That time period is a key part of this fascinating correlation: infant colic emerges a few days after birth—at about the same time that the residual progesterone (from the mother's body) is being excreted in the urine of the baby. Endocrinologists have found that some infants begin to produce their own progesterone within forty-eight hours of birth, while in others no evidence of progesterone can be found for several months. Bradford and his coauthors theorized that this difference among infants "might constitute a lag period during which the colic infants are without a muscle-relaxing hormone."

The researchers conducted a series of chemical analyses on the urine of fifteen newborns without colic and eight newborns with colic. The non-colicky children were ten males and five females ranging in age from six days to three months; none developed colic at any time. The urine of all fifteen contained pregnanediol, which physicians use as a measure of the circulating progesterone in the body.

Then the researchers conducted the same chemical analysis on the urine of eight colicky babies—three males and five females ranging in age from two to ten weeks. They found no pregnanediol in the urine of five of the infants, and in the other three the hormone was "just barely visible" and tended to fade out after a few minutes on the chemically treated paper prepared to measure it.

The researchers then tested a third group of seven colicky children by measuring the pregnanediol in their urine, giving them small oral doses of progesterone and measuring their pregnanediol levels again, while observing their colic symptoms. The children were four males and three females, ranging in age from four to eleven weeks.

In each of the seven colicky children the first chemical test showed no pregnanediol in their urine. The colic symptoms were described as "moderate" in five and "severe" in two. Following the oral administration of small amounts of progesterone, the urine of all seven contained pregnanediol. One child was then characterized as "less fussy"; five were described as "improved"; and one was termed "much better."

The authors surmised that "whereas in the noncolic infant . . . progesterone serves to sustain a muscle-relaxing activity, in the colic infant this fetal response is absent or delayed" because the colicky infants have not yet begun to manufacture their own progesterone.

The 1963 research was not taken as conclusive, because the number of children involved was small. More important, the side effects and long-term consequences of hormone therapy are not well understood, and doctors are reluctant to embrace so drastic a measure for a condition as limited as colic. One endocrinologist said in an interview, "There are many better ways of handling colic than with a hormone. If progesterone was the *only* remedy available, you can be sure the drug companies would have developed it."

The most mystifying fact of colic behavior is that colicky babies who are born prematurely don't develop their colic symptoms until full-term babies do—that is, until the premature infant is a week or two past its full-term due date. If colic is a developmental problem, then logically premature newborns should have a much higher rate of colic, and they would develop the symptoms almost immediately after birth. But neither is the case.

In 1948 Dr. Paul P. Pierce observed a number of premature infants at the Rochester Child Health Project in Rochester, Minn. In those who developed colic, he wrote, "the onset was delayed for a period approximately in proportion to their degree of prematurity." Pierce emphasized that the behavior of the cases he observed could not have been explained on the basis of improper feeding technique or hunger. His belief was that a developmental factor contributed to the cause of the colic, and that the factor "may primarily be related to the state or maturity of some part of the nervous system." The obvious question then is, must newborns reach a certain level of maturity or development *before* colic symptoms can emerge? No study has yet provided an answer.

Dr. Jack Paradise in his 1966 colic report suggested that new insights into the causes of colic "might be gained from additional study of infants' responses to swaddling, rhythmic motion and vibration." He was intrigued by the possibility that colic "is an expression of central nervous system immaturity." If so, he wrote, "colic may be viewed as a normal maturational phenomenon." The things that often tend to soothe colicky infants—sucking, swaddling, rocking, monotonous noise or vibration—may "work" because they interrupt certain nerve impulses or stimuli traveling from the infant's belly to its brain.

Many researchers have mentioned "central nervous system immaturity" as a possible cause of colic. It is entirely logical that the nerve systems that control the activity of the intestines are not functioning smoothly in the first weeks of life in some infants. Research has established that the infant's heartbeat is irregular for many weeks after birth; simple observation tells parents that the newborn's breathing is uneven. The baby's brand-new muscles and nerves haven't settled into a rhythm yet, and this is not exceptional—it is the norm for virtually all newborns.

Since we know that in the early weeks of life all these nerve systems haven't got their signals straight yet in terms of the infant's breathing and heartbeat, it is not too speculative to believe that in some infants the same irregularities exist between the central nervous system and the muscles of the intestines. Thus the intestines may be working unevenly, with slight spasms, just as the heart does.

Some medications that have been occasionally effective for colic are "parasympathetic depressors"—that is, they depress the impulses of the parasympathetic nerves (the "autonomic" or self-controlling nerve systems such as those that regulate the muscle functions of peristalsis, the contractions that move food through the intestines), and thus leave the intestines more relaxed and less prone to spasms.

It is also possible that these uneven and irregular nerve signals can be interrupted or smoothed out by some other stimulation—motion, vibration, warmth, or low-level monotonous noise. Just as adults find certain external stimulation very soothing—the sound of falling rain, the beating of waves on a beach—perhaps the infant's "jittery" nerve system can be calmed by the ticking of a clock, gentle rocking, the vibration of a moving car, or an automatic baby swing. We think of these "tricks" as distracting the baby from its discomfort; in fact, they may do more: they may help settle the rhythm of a newborn's jumpy and immature nerve system.

Perhaps the only research relating infant irritability to the central nervous system is in the area of swaddling. In the 1960s Dr. Earle Lipton and others published a series of studies reporting their extensive research on the practice of swaddling and its physiological effect on babies. Swaddling is the ancient practice, common in many cultures, of wrapping infants in lengths of cloth and thus severely restricting the movement of the infant's legs, arms, and torso.

In a 1965 supplement to *Pediatrics*, Lipton and his coauthors acknowledged the work of a researcher who "induced sleep in young infants by restraining them in his arms, often rocking and singing to them and closing their eyelids with his fingers." They found that "increased sleeping, less crying, and lowered respiratory and cardiac rates" generally resulted from swaddling.

Lipton and his colleagues found experimental support for the hypothesis that restraint of motor activity by itself has a quieting effect on infants, and they wrote, "We have been impressed by the results [of swaddling] in several cases of irritability in young infants." But the connection between a practice like swaddling and the functioning of the central nervous system remains conjectural and circumstantial at best.

To confuse matters further, a 1971 report in the *American Journal of the Diseases of Children* discounted central nervous system immaturity as a cause of colic, based on a study of infants having a low birth weight. The authors, John E. Meyer and Dr. M. Michael Thaler of San Francisco, wrote that they had surveyed the infants "to determine whether developmental immaturity or intrauterine growth retardation plays a role" in the development of colic.

They examined the birth records of 262 infants born at a San Francisco hospital between 1963 and 1967 with a birth weight of five pounds, eight ounces or less. They identified colic in 11.4 percent of the infants, but could find no correlation of the colic to the newborn's sex, birth weight, birth order, gestational age, or perinatal factors such as a difficult birth, breast- or bottle-feeding, and so on.

Because the incidence of colic among infants of low birth weight was within the statistical range reported by Paradise (who studied full-term children) and was identical to the incidence (11.6 percent) observed by the same authors in a separate study of full-term babies, Meyer and Thaler wrote that "neither gestational immaturity nor intra uterine growth retardation appears to carry a predisposition to colic." And that being the case, they concluded, "these findings weaken the possibility that colic represents an immaturity of the central nervous system."

Certainly these conditions in the infant's plumbing hold a great potential for the understanding and treatment of colic—enzyme efficiency, progesterone levels, intestinal spasm caused either by a progesterone deficiency or by irregular nerve impulses in an immature central nervous system. Unfortunately they are also fairly technical areas of physiology and development, and research into these factors would require sophisticated techniques carried out under carefully controlled circumstances. Further knowledge in this field—even when it is developed in the laboratory—is not likely to filter down quickly, in a useable form, to the pediatrician and the parent.

But on the chance that the theories of central nervous

system immaturity are correct—or correct for even a few infants—you should try the tactics that might impose order on your baby's unsettled system: rhythmic motion, monotonous noise, or swaddling. If you try swaddling, be sure to discuss the idea with your pediatrician to be certain you will not make the baby too hot or bind it too tightly.

Medications: Sometimes a Comfort, But Never a Cure

The medications commonly in use today for infant colic include mild sedatives, which in small doses allow the infant to sleep through its discomfort, and—just as important—allow the parent a period of recovery; preparations that can break up and disperse some of the gas in the child's system; and drugs that act on the nerve systems of the intestines to relax spastic muscle activity there.

Pediatricians today are far more reluctant than they ever were to prescribe medications—particularly for conditions where the drug can't effect a "cure." Thus it is often the parent who pressures the physician for a medication: "Isn't there something you can *give* the baby?"

Physicians tended to "give something" as much to soothe the parent as the child, until research evidence began to accumulate that what they were giving had little effect on the colic, but might have undesirable side effects. That, in fact, is the history of the search for medications that can be applied safely to infant colic.

In 1940 a University of Kansas pediatrician was a leading advocate of the use of sedatives in the treatment of colic symptoms. Dr. Frank C. Neff wrote in the *Journal of the American Medical Association* that the newborn arriving home from the hospital encounters harsh stimulation almost too extensive to list, "the chief being the doorbell, the radio, the telephone, the activities of various members of the household, the visits of friends, the many services from tradesmen, and the street noises."

Neff maintained that the screaming of some infants was an extension of the startle reflex.* His remedy for this was the most soothing environment possible. "It is well to avoid unnecessary handling," he wrote. "A minimum of attention directed by adults toward this infant will quiet the condition." Not many parents today would agree that the treatment of colic is so easy, and perhaps the "minimum of attention" strategy is a greater boon to the haggard parent than to the crying infant. (Obviously, the success of many colic "remedies" is judged by how much they help the *parents.*) Many parents find they simply *cannot* let the colicky infant cry by itself, even after they've decided to try Neff's strategy. And for normal development, babies need a certain level of social interaction with their parents . . . even if—for the duration of the colic—the interaction seems unsatisfying to both parents and child.

Neff recommended mild doses of any of four medications—paregoric, phenobarbital, atropine, and codeine—all of which are viewed with misgiving by parents and pediatricians today. Both codeine and paregoric have narcotic side effects; they "drug" the infant into drowsiness and dull its senses. Atropine is used to relax the smooth muscles in various body organs, but a common side effect is the fever it induces ("atropine fever") in children taking the drug. Phenobarbital may be the least objectionable of the sedative drugs; its effect is to counter muscle spasms, but it also keeps children in a sleepy and

* Startle reflex: the involuntary jump or movement of an infant as a reaction to a sudden stimulation like noise or touch.

lethargic state . . . not a condition that encourages normal development.

In journal articles in the mid-1950s the Swedish researcher Sigvard Jorup and the English researcher R. S. Illingworth debated the value of a drug called skopyl for relieving colic pains. Skopyl (methylscopolamine nitrate) was the short name given to an antispasmodic drug—that is, one intended to prevent spasms in the colon. Jorup praised the medication highly in his studies of 111 "dyspeptic" breast-fed infants.

"Dyspepsia" is an impairment of the power or function of digestion—the term is often applied to abdominal pain following meals. Jorup had investigated the frequency and nature of dyspepsia in infants he called "neurolabile" —those with unstable nervous systems.

Of 589 children his study examined at a child welfare center in Stockholm, Jorup found 30 percent with the digestive problem he called dyspepsia. The dyspeptic children's X rays showed a "convulsively contracted colon" and "a propulsive motility of the colon on feeding." These propulsive contractions moved food through the colon too quickly; thus fluids were not properly absorbed into the body, and—the fluids remaining with the food—the result was diarrhea. Jorup wrote that "it was possible to induce the propulsive motility of the colon by giving either breast milk or cow's milk mixtures by different means, and on some occasions by the mere act of sucking."

Jorup called the "propulsive motility" of the colon hyperperistalsis—that is, an overactive motion of the muscles in the intestines. He turned to skopyl as an antispasmodic medication and found that it "produced a rapid effect on the loose stools and attacks of pain"—in other words, that it relaxed the propulsive contractions, slowed down the passage of food, and allowed a greater absorption of fluids into the body.

Among his 111 dyspeptic subjects, Jorup was emphatic in his belief that "the majority of cases of so-called three-months colic are attributable" to the hyperperistalsis that he blamed for dyspepsia. It is possible, however, that the value of the medication as an antispasmodic for intestinal spasms was independent of its resolution of diarrhea. Modern studies conclude that diarrhea is neither a cause nor a result of colic. A colicky infant can have diarrhea, however, and in such cases the parents' work with a pediatrician to end the diarrhea may improve the baby's digestion of food and somewhat ease its discomfort.

Illingworth disagreed about the value of skopyl. At the Jessop Hospital for Women in Sheffield, England, he instituted an eighteen-month study with forty infants having moderate or severe colic. He divided the infants into two groups of twenty: one group would get a mild "control substance" (ascorbic acid*) for comparison purposes, while the other group was given skopyl as an antispasmodic "in the dosage recommended by the makers . . . four times a day . . . before feeds." There were no significant differences between the two groups, although the weekly weight gain was slightly higher among the infants in the group given skopyl. Sixteen of the twenty babies in each group were fully breast-fed. The average duration of treatment in both groups was about eighteen days.

Five infants in the skopyl group and nine in the control group were judged to be "much better or cured" with the substance given them. Nine babies in the skopyl group and seven in the control group were found to be "better." One child in the skopyl group was found to be "worse" and four in the skopyl group were "much worse," compared to none in each category in the control group.

Illingworth concluded that skopyl used in the dosage

* Ascorbic acid: Vitamin C, essential for normal metabolism.

recommended by the makers was of no value in the treatment of colic. He cautioned, "In a self-limiting condition . . . it is easy to give a drug credit for curing a patient when in fact it has achieved nothing." An antispasmodic drug, skopyl is a derivative of atropine, and Illingworth warned against its use in outpatient situations "because of the danger of toxic reactions."

Four years later, in 1959, Illingworth decided to evaluate a new medication with the commercial name Merbentyl®. With fewer side effects, Merbentyl (dicyclomine hydrochloride) acted to depress the parasympathetic nerves. In this research Illingworth used the "double-blind" method of testing the medication on his forty colicky subjects. In the double-blind method the test drug is used along with a control substance—an inert material for comparison purposes—but someone *other* than the researcher keeps the records that tell which infants are getting which substance. The method rules out expectations by the researcher or the parents that might influence the results. In this case the chief pharmacist of Jessop Hospital dispensed the drug and kept the records, so both Illingworth and the infants' parents were "blind" to which substance the babies were getting. The pharmacist dispensed either the drug or an inert substance and Illingworth saw the child a week later and recorded what the mother said about the colic. During the following week the pharmacist gave the opposite of what she had given before.

On each visit Illingworth "scored" the results for each child from −3, meaning the child was much worse, to +3, meaning the child was much better and free of symptoms. By this method Merbentyl "outscored" the inert comparison substance: the mothers rated the drug at +47, and the inert substance at +19—that is, they reported a definite improvement with the Merbentyl.

Illingworth was convinced. He wrote that his study "has proved that the drug is of considerable value." The drug acted to "block" the nerves that activate certain muscles in the intestine. Marketed as Merbentyl in England and Bentyl® in the United States, the drug is available for infant colic, although pediatricians in the last few years have backed away from *all* medications in unharmful and self-limiting conditions like colic. One pediatrician explained, "Like everything else, it works for the first day. Other than that, I haven't had any real success with it." A derivative is sometimes still used to treat the severe contractions of pylorospasm.

The best recent evaluation of the use of medications for colic was reported in the October 1979 issue of the *American Journal of the Diseases of Childhood*, in an article reporting research on ninety-seven colicky infants over a five-year period, conducted in Baltimore, Md., by a pediatrician and a pharmacist, J. C. O'Donovan, M.D., and A. S. Bradstock, Jr. They evaluated two common colic preparations—phenobarbital in an alcohol solution, and phenobarbital and homatropine methylbromide in an alcohol solution. As control substances, they added to their study an alcohol solution alone, and a "placebo" solution —water with artificial coloring.

This research, too, was double-blind. No other medications were prescribed, but the parents of all ninety-seven babies were given as much support as possible, and were encouraged to try formula changes, car rides, wind-up swings, and so on, to relieve their babies' colic pains.

The research actually found that of the children who were improved or cured, sixteen had been taking the placebo (colored water) solution, while eighteen had been taking the phenobarbital solution and eighteen the phenobarbital and homatropine methylbromide solution. In fact, of the children taking the nonmedicinal placebo (the colored water), 84 percent were improved or cured; but of the children taking the phenobarbital-homatropine solution, 70 percent were improved or cured. And of those taking the phenobarbital and alcohol solution, 67 percent were improved or cured. Thus, neither of the two medicinal solutions improved or cured a greater percentage of the children than the water placebo did.

The study also measured the duration of the infants' colic attacks during the treatment period. Of the children who showed no improvement, substantially more were taking the phenobarbital-homatropine solution than the placebo. Of those who were improved, the percentage taking the placebo was nearly as great as the percentage taking the phenobarbital-homatropine preparation. And of those whose crying was completely resolved, a far greater percentage were taking the placebo than were taking either the phenobarbital alone or in combination with homatropine methylbromide.

"Of the drugs studied, none was more [effective] than a placebo," the researchers wrote, and they concluded that "neither alcohol, phenobarbital, nor homatropine are of value in the therapy of colic." Significantly, just after the study ended, the manufacturer notified physicians that the homatropine methylbromide compound would be removed from Sedadrops®—probably the most widely used medication for colic in the United States at that time—and that infant colic was being dropped from the list of appropriate usages for Sedadrops.

Like so many other colic "remedies," the effectiveness of Sedadrops was a sometime thing, even before the compound was altered and no longer recommended for colic. Some mothers reported that the drug helped their infants' colic symptoms, and other parents said that it had no effect. In that respect, Sedadrops was no different from virtually all other therapies that have been applied to infant colic. In their article, O'Donovan and Bradstock wrote, "The principal unanswered question remains, 'What are you treating when you treat colic?' " And they were emphatic—but not alone—in their answer: "We believe colic is a heterogeneous entity and not one condition at all."

Terrific. The questions seem to get broader rather than narrower. That's one of the problems with research: it sometimes seems that the more you know, the more confused you are. Perhaps we should ask: has research benefited the family with a colicky infant?

The Bottom Line: Has Research Helped the Parent?

Absolutely.

There is simply no doubt that even with its gaps and contradictions, medical research has vastly improved our ability to cope with colic. For one thing, the knowledge gained from research has given us confidence—confidence, often, to follow our instincts and do what we feel we ought to be doing. And because confidence is a large part of getting through the baby's colicky period, it is probably fair to say that the research knowledge has helped parents (by relieving their anxieties) more than it has helped the infants (by relieving their discomfort).

Let's review the major areas of research knowledge that we can use in coping with colic.

First of all, research has told us what colic is *not*. Infant colic bears absolutely no relationship to the baby's sex or birth order, the mother's age or illnesses during pregnancy, the term of her pregnancy or the race and blood type of the mother and infant, the mother's weight gain during pregnancy or the baby's weight gain after birth, the style of childbirth or the drugs administered to the mother during labor and delivery. Colic is unrelated to fetal hiccups, the mother's choice of breast milk or bottle formula, the family's socioeconomic status, other gastrointestinal symptoms in the infant, or an excessive amount of gas in the baby's system. And research has found no correlation between infant colic and vomiting, diarrhea, constipation, the number of bowel movements daily, convulsions, or breath-holding.

The list of factors that colic *does* correlate with is a great deal shorter: one researcher found that colicky crying increases with the duration of the feeding. Others found that a high ratio of colicky children have older brothers and sisters who had colic as infants. And although several major studies insist that allergies are not a part of colic, too many unresolved questions remain about the relationship of colic to allergies.

In England thirty years ago X-ray procedures were carried out on a small number of severely colicky children as part of a larger study of colic. In none of the children could X-ray evidence be found of excessive internal gas. This led the researcher to conclude that the problem is in the *passage* of a normal amount of gas—that is, a spasm or kinking traps gas in the intestine.

From research studies centering on how allergies *do* seem to relate to colic we learn that a family history of allergies seems to occur often in the families of colicky children—though no one can say why. We learn that a lactose intolerance to cow's milk (which medical research shows is far higher among blacks than among whites) is different from colic, because it can fairly easily be discovered and remedied. And we learn that both researchers and nursing mothers have reported that foods eaten by the mother can be transmitted through breast milk, resulting in colicky behavior in the nursing infant. Eggs seem to be the commonest offender.

Another type of research knowledge, chemical in nature, is interesting because it is puzzling and—sad to say—not yet very useful in the daily confrontation between parents and colic. In testing the urine of colicky children, researchers failed to find evidence of a "normal" supply of progesterone, a hormone that helps to control the muscle activity of some internal organs. This and subsequent tests led researchers to the conclusion that colicky infants temporarily lack a sufficient supply of progesterone, and consequently their stomach and intestinal muscles may cramp spasmodically. Another possible cause of colic is a deficiency of enzymes in the gastric juices of the stomach. This temporary enzyme shortage may make it difficult for some infants to break down and digest their food—particularly carbohydrates and butterfats.

The theories of colic take on more meaning for parents when researchers manipulate various factors to try to identify and eliminate the causes of infant colic. The symptoms of colic have shown improvement when the duration of feedings was shortened and infants were kept in a semi-inclined posture during and after feedings; when carbohydrates and butterfats were eliminated from bottle formulas and when nursing mothers eliminated eggs, cow's milk, and other foods from their own diets; when infants were given thicker feedings or offered a pacifier between meals; and when the number of daily feedings was increased and the amount of each feeding was reduced.

Recent research has shown medications to be generally ineffective as a remedy for colic. Some of the older drugs are now regarded as simply too potent for infants, and too likely to produce undesirable side effects. Other drugs have been altered by their manufacturers and are no longer recommended for colic. Only in the most extreme cases will physicians today prescribe a medication for colic: usually a gas-dispersing agent, or a very mild sedative.

Finally, recent research fails to support the notion that family tension and maternal anxiety can cause infant colic, although few would dispute the idea that "situational stress" can worsen the infant/family interaction and make the colic far harder to tolerate.

Despite these findings, we may not know all the causes of infant colic. But even apart from allergies and milk intolerance, we can identify five possible causes: too much food at a single feeding, causing pain as contractions of the stomach and small intestine attempt to force food through the digestive system; too few enzymes in the infant's stomach, making it difficult for the baby to break down and digest carbohydrates and butterfats; too little progesterone in the infant's hormonal production, leading to spasms in the intestines; intestinal spasms and kinking, which magnify the discomfort of trapped gas; and an undeveloped central nervous system, causing spasms in the digestive system and sending painful stimuli to the brain. All the research reviewed here points to specific steps parents can take to try to relieve their infant's colic.

These steps begin with the elimination of all potentially allergenic foods from the baby's diet—notably butterfats, carbohydrates, and cow's milk—and the elimination of milk, eggs, and other troublesome foods from the nursing mother's diet. Parents' efforts may also include the "low stimulation" home environment suggested by Neff, and a concerted attack (with the help of the pediatrician) on diarrhea if that accompanies the baby's colic.

Tactics will include special attention to feeding techniques and burping, and calming the infant's nervous system with rhythmic motion, monotonous noise, or swaddling. You may be able to help your baby pass gas by changing its posture or gently massaging its belly. You may also apply Brackett's theory of feeding smaller amounts at more frequent intervals, and you will want to find out if a pacifier will comfort the child.

Finally, for your own sake, put out of your mind the fear that your own tension or anxiety have somehow caused the baby's colic. Any technique that will help *you* relax—a glass of wine, soothing music, or a walk in the park—will help you cope with the baby's colicky behavior, so pay attention to your own needs as well.

At the very least, the research that led to these conclusions has made colic less mysterious and more understandable.

THREE

Parents and Pediatricians

Typically, when mother and baby arrive home from the hospital, everything seems just fine for a few days . . . even if the baby does seem a little fussy at first. Over the next week or two—if you are like most "colic parents" I encountered—the excitement of telephone calls and baby gifts gave way to the realization that when the baby wasn't sleeping or feeding, it was crying.

And not just crying, either, but *screaming* . . . with an intensity you'd never seen in friends' children. In many cases the infant's whole body twists as the baby kicks and struggles, its face turning red and contorted. Worst of all, you couldn't comfort the baby in any of the time-honored ways: carrying and patting, rocking and humming, changing diapers or nursing or playing with a rattle.

That was when your first real concerns started: with the realization that no matter what you did—distractions, walks, cuddling, rocking—the shrieking would go on and on . . . through mealtimes, when the baby was alone in its crib, and when you were trying to talk to other people, no matter who was holding it, during nap times and late into the night when everyone else in the family was exhausted.

After a week of trying to remain calm and deliberate about the agonized screaming, your growing alarm forced the decision: at what point should you call the pediatrician?

When to Call the Doctor

Concern and worry about the baby's crying are legitimate reasons for calling the doctor. In fact, pediatricians expect parents to call under such circumstances. "The call itself indicates a genuine problem," explains Meade Christian, a North Carolina pediatrician. "Parents won't call unless they're very worried and frustrated." Christian approaches colic as "a problem for parents." He's the one who said, "I know the *kid* is going to make it. My orientation is toward the parents."

Physicians know that the fatigue, anxiety, and frustration that accumulate over a period of weeks have the potential to cause dangerous problems in some families. One pediatrician said, "I don't think a bad case of infant colic can harm a stable marriage. But where there are already latent problems—marriage tensions, alcohol problems, financial stress—severe colic can push some couples beyond their endurance, and then you're dealing with the possibility of abuse or violence. I tell parents, 'You've got to call me when you feel you just can't stand it anymore.' " All of the doctors interviewed tend to regard the severity of the colic not in terms of the infant's discomfort, but of the impact on the family.

No responsible physician will offer advice to parents without first examining the child. Dr. James L. Dennis, former director of Children's Hospital in Oakland, Calif., has been quoted as saying, "I believe in an old adage: 'For each mistake made for not knowing, ten are made for not looking.' I want to examine a baby before deciding he has colic."

The Imperative of the Physical Exam

Dr. Harold Meyer, associate executive director of the American Board of Pediatrics, Inc., described some of the information doctors will want to know when parents first bring in a colicky infant:

> *The physician will usually want a detailed history that may go all the way back to the planning of the conception, and the history of the pregnancy. Did the mother take medications during her pregnancy, and was her labor difficult or prolonged? He wants to know the mother's perception of how the baby behaves, sleeps and feeds. Because the mother-infant bonding may be very tentative and fragile at first, the doctor will want to* see *the mother-infant interaction. He'll want to know what kind of family support structures exist at home, particularly the father's help and feelings. Finally he'll want to know the child's dietary history—is the baby bottlefed or breastfed? This background information helps the physician do a sensible physical examination of the baby.*

Most physicians regard the diagnosis of infant colic as a process of exclusion. "It's not difficult," says Dr. Jim Schwankle, a pediatrician with practices in two rural communities. "It's a matter of ruling out organic causes and then working on the others." Because colic is so variable in its possible causes from child to child, Dr. Ambrose McGee of Virginia characterized the process as an attempt "to find the rule to fit the child."

In ruling out the organic causes, how do physicians satisfy themselves that the symptoms don't indicate something more serious than colic?

"I look at the growth chart first," says Dr. Meade Christian. "The baby's gains in weight and length are very sensitive indicators of whether or not there's an organic problem. When I talk to the parents I try to determine whether there's a colic pattern—the time of day when the crying is worst, the baby's behavior, and so on. My physical exam looks for things like ear infection and hernia. And I tell the parents a few things to watch out for at home." For example, Christian wants the parents to observe the baby's appetite and the regularity of its bowel movements, and to watch out for fever, congestion or breathing difficulty, severe vomiting, or dehydration.

The physical exam must rule out factors like milk intolerance, which often is indicated by allergic reactions such as eczema, diarrhea, and regurgitating. Coliclike symptoms are also produced by a condition known as intussesception, in which one part of the intestine folds or slips inside an adjacent part, rather like the fit of a smaller end of pipe or hose inside a larger end. But this condition is very unusual.

Diagnosing Infant Colic

In a 1976 article in the *Canadian Medical Association Journal*, Dr. Joseph N. H. Du warned his colleagues that urinary tract infection can present many of the same initial symptoms as colic. Dr. Du noted that in four years of carefully evaluating many infants with colic, he had discovered four cases of urinary tract infection, three of which responded quickly to prescription medications. He recommended urologic examination of infants with "severe intractable colic" that persisted for more than three months despite proper management.

A 1944 article by Dr. Benjamin Spock in the journal *Psychosomatic Medicine* drew the distinction between infant colic and pyloric stenosis, a condition far more serious than but very smilar to colic in the baby's crying behavior. Pyloric stenosis, Spock wrote, "commonly produces its symptoms several weeks after birth. There is perisistent projectile vomiting which leads to dehydration, constipation, and emaciation."

Organically, pyloric stenosis is a condition in which the circular muscle of the pyloric valve, from the stomach to the intestine, becomes enlarged in a way that completely closes the sphincter and obstructs the passage of food. The condition is not common (it occurs in only about 0.5 percent of all births in this country) but it is dangerous, and often the only successful treatment will involve surgery.

Spock reviewed previous research that concluded that pyloric stenosis occurred more often in male infants, in firstborn children, and among twins; and that it may have a multiple incidence in some families, occurring in two, three, or four children.

In a 1938 article in the *Virginia Medical Monthly*, Dr. Eugene Keiter discussed a number of other conditions that must be taken into account in diagnosing infant colic, such as acute respiratory infections, which can normally be seen and heard, and other infections, which are usually accompanied by fever. The rarer causes of coliclike symptoms include congenital syphilis, bone fractures that might have occurred in an exceptionally difficult delivery, appendicitis, hernia, or volvulous (an obstruction resulting from a knotting or twisting in the intestine). Keiter noted that colic spasms pass without ill effects, whereas most of the rare and more serious conditions become steadily worse over a period of hours, thus making diagnosis more certain.

Once the physical examination has confirmed the diagnosis of infant colic, how does the pediatrician approach the treatment of the condition in discussing it with parents?

"I start by telling parents that colic is a syndrome of behaviors," says Dr. Schwankle. "I almost never assign a particular cause to the condition, because then something gets 'blamed' to the exclusion of all the other factors involved, and I don't believe that is realistic or effective."

Dr. Christian concurs. "I tell parents that colic is a descriptive term of behavior. I tell them that their baby is not sick—parents need to hear that. But not everyone can use that information to get through. My job then is to relieve any guilt the parents might feel that they are doing something wrong, and to help them work out a plan for how they are going to deal with it."

Clearly the professional opinion changes often, and physicians themselves have worries about the helpfulness of the advice they give. Dr. Carl A. Holmes, writing in the journal *Clinical Pediatrics*, observed that the fact that "colic occurs most often late at night, whereas most babies are seen by the doctor in the daytime, may help to explain why many doctors do not look upon colic as a serious entity."

Holmes may have overstated the case—most pediatricians now do understand how difficult infant colic can be for parents to endure. But it is a fact that when parents get desperate enough to call their pediatrician and make an appointment, they want the doctor to see a *colicky* child. Nothing is more infuriating to parents than to carry a colicky infant and a half-ton of paraphernalia to the pediatrician's office, only to have the baby lie quietly on its back playing with its toes and gurgling cutely at the doctor. The parents feel like idiots.

If your child's colic is in fact worse late in the day, you may not want a doctor's appointment at nine-thirty in the morning. Secretly, most parents want the baby to put on a real show, so a four-thirty afternoon appointment may be the best. The physician may not appreciate the screaming at the end of his or her *own* tiring day, but at least you will feel you are getting your money's worth out of the visit if the doctor sees what you must put up with at home.

When parents turn to the pediatrician for help with a colicky baby, they are in part seeking medical help and information ("You want answers," said one mother; "you want an explanation . . .") and in part seeking encouragement and understanding. Dr. Clifford David observes, "Sometimes when parents reach a certain point of frustration and exhaustion, they need your professional blessing that they can do *less*. If the infant is dry, well fed, comfortable and safe, and still screaming, the parent must know that it's permissible to put the baby down, leave the room, and shut the door. When you've done everything you humanly can, there's nothing wrong with doing *nothing*." Pediatrician Robert Brownlee agrees that this is one of the hardest ideas for parents to acknowledge and act upon. "You're no help to the child, no help to your mate, and you can't expect to cope very effectively when you're fatigued and overstressed," he says.

As a matter of perspective, the parents of colicky children must keep in mind that there is considerable evidence that infant colic is less common—or less commonly reported—in many cultures around the world. The notion of "going to the doctor" for a condition that is not an outright emergency is—to put it bluntly—a luxury of middle-class societies. In order for a condition like infant colic to come to the attention of doctors, physicians must be: (1) very numerous; (2) very accessible, in terms of time and distance; (3) not preoccupied with saving the lives of starving children; (4) financially affordable, in those countries where the private medical practice is the common form of health care; and (5) it must be socially acceptable to use physicians for routine complaints where a life is not in danger.

For example, Dr. Alan Cross recalls that in his experience in East Africa, where infants are at risk of dying of malnutrition, pneumonia, and age-old diseases, "colic was never mentioned, nor—in two years—did any parent bring in a child with a complaint that might be classified as colic."

Dr. Brian Connor, an Australian physician, had the same experience: "This does not mean to say that there was no such thing as colic, but that it never was considered something to see the doctors about." Connor also noted that in societies where the extended family is still close by, a harassed mother has more help and relief. And he thought that the more primitive pattern of nearly constant breast-feeding was probably easier on infants' digestion: "I don't believe the human baby is made to have large feeds at infrequent and irregular intervals (often geared to the clock or family arrangements)."

In some developing countries where these ancient family patterns are changing, colic may emerge as a more commonly encountered problem. Dr. Clifford David, for example, practiced pediatrics in San'a, the capital of Yemen. "More and more, the young men come into the cities from the remote villages to find jobs," he observed. "When they begin to earn money, they return to the village, marry, and bring their wives back to the city. So, many young couples are somewhat alone—far from their families

—and a little disoriented—at a time in their lives when they begin to have children."

In Japan, another family-centered society, very few pediatricians have even *heard* of infant colic. This sounds at first like a terrific advertisement for Japanese life-style and diet—indeed, both factors may contribute to the low reported rate of colic in Japan. But another factor is at work, too, and that is the structure of well-baby care in the Japanese medical system. Normally, a Japanese infant will not even have a first well-baby checkup until the age of three months—that is, about the time that colic ends. A sick child, of course, would be taken to a pediatrician before that. But without some overt sign of illness, most Japanese newborns are not seen by medical professionals until they are about twelve weeks old.

Dr. Hugh J. Heggerty, pediatrician at the Child Development Centre at York District Hospital in England, admits his frustration in pinpointing just what infant colic is, what causes it, and how to resolve it: "In very few of my patients have we reached some explanation as to the reason for [colic] pain . . . I must admit that of all the children I see with this complaint very, very few ever reach a certain diagnostic conclusion."

That colic is a genuine physical malady is unquestionable. But the fact that 15 to 20 percent of all American newborns need a physician's attention because of colic may be a reflection of our casual access to medical care rather than a measure of the severity of the condition itself.

It seems clear that most American pediatricians would rather be relied on as resources for support than as pill-prescribers. Still, the parent is the one who is at home with the screaming infant, day in and day out, week after week. How do you get through it? To gain confidence in your approach it's logical to ask: How did others cope?

FOUR

Coping with Colic

"I had plenty of people giving me advice and telling me they hadn't seen anything like it," a mother of a colicky girl reported. "But mostly, it was just me and my husband."

It may be hard to keep in mind, but grandparents, in-laws, and friends may be just as confounded by your baby's colicky behavior as you are. The interviews conducted for this book, however, led to two unexpected conclusions: first, friends and family are probably a direct help to the parents of colicky babies in more cases than one would have guessed was possible; second, the parents of colicky infants are better than expected at accepting such help.

But there are problems. In our mobile society families with young children often do not live near enough to the grandparents to get sustained support from them. And many mothers at home with young infants find that their friends and even their parents are at work during the day, and unavailable to help.

"My mother was nearby, but she worked," said a woman with premature colicky twins—her husband was on rotating shifts at the police department—"and my grandmother really couldn't do much except offer a lot of encouragement."

"My parents both worked," another woman said, "and I felt we got minimal encouragement from family and doctors. But a neighbor helped, to talk to, and my husband was the best support."

"I talked a great deal to other mothers in church, from our Lamaze class, and in the La Leche League," one mother recalled. And if it is possible to have a colicky child and be lucky, there was the woman who reported, "I relied on live-in help. We hired someone to get the older kids out of the house, and to let me get out."

A few mothers reported that their friends were not very helpful, for a variety of understandable reasons. (One factor lies in the perception of the person needing help—in an experience as intense as infant colic, it often seems to the parents that "no one really understands what we're going through.") One mother reported that when her infant daughter was colicky, "I was twenty-three and few of my friends had children yet, so they couldn't really appreciate what I needed."

At the other end of the childbearing years: "My friends were older and not having babies any longer," a former Michigan resident explained. "My husband was in medical school and although my mom came, she stayed only a week." Another woman remembers, "I felt cut off. . . . My friends were involved in other things and not interested in my problem."

In the interviews with parents there were only a few horror stories. One was the woman who blamed her grandchild's colic on her daughter-in-law's nursing. Another was the woman who told a Massachusetts mother of a colicky boy, "You wanted a girl, that's why you don't like him." (In ordinary circumstances, most parents can dismiss such thoughtless remarks with a good laugh, but infant colic is no ordinary circumstance, and such witless comments can send worried, vulnerable parents into weeks of self-doubt: "Did I *really* want a girl that badly?") Overall, such stories stand out only because there are so few of them.

The grandparents and in-laws we heard about were almost invariably sympathetic and supportive. "My mother gave me a great deal of advice and encouragement," another Massachusetts mother said. And a South Carolina woman recalled, "My mother-in-law helped a lot during the first six weeks. At least we could get away."

But because in our society friends are often geographically closer than family, the parents of colicky children frequently find themselves relying on friends and neighbors.

- "Friends baby-sat for us, even though I was reluctant to go out," reported an Indiana woman whose daughter's colic lasted nearly four months.
- "My mother was with us for two weeks after our little boy was born, and everything was wonderful," another woman said. "Then on the day she left he started screaming and doubling up from seven P.M. to midnight. At first we thought he missed her. We had just moved to town, none of our new friends had kids yet, and we wouldn't have known where to go if we *did* get out. But one friend did come over and rocked the baby to give me a break. It really helped."
- One parent reported, "Our families were too far away when our daughter was born, but I had one close friend, about ten years

older than me, and I called her every two or three days for four months."

- "A girl friend of mine also had a colicky baby at about the same time," a North Carolina woman remembered, "so we traded advice and suggestions."
- A mother whose sixth child was colicky said, "I got some help from my grandmother and a neighbor, but mostly, my older kids were big enough by then to help out."
- And a New England mother whose infant son was colicky for four months said, "A close friend of mine would walk with me outdoors, or come in and hold him while I napped."

These one-hour breaks or catnaps may seem inconsequential, but even a short respite can help an overstressed mother rejuvenate herself. Even the most helpful friends, however, can't provide the professional reassurance that parents seek from a pediatrician. In helping the parents cope with colic, what does the physician do, as parents see it? And what is the parents' perception of the results?

How Much Can the Doctor Really Help?

"Our doctor didn't give us any remedy for the colic," a New England mother said. "He said he'd give *me* some tranquilizers if I asked for them."

And another woman said, "With our first colicky baby we didn't really have a regular physician; with our second, I knew what to expect and I don't think I ever asked for a doctor's help."

Many pediatricians—but not all—now believe that since the treatment of the colicky baby is very limited (mostly to diet manipulations), the best they can do is treat the parents' anxiety and concerns. This does not mean that modern pediatricians will ignore the baby's discomfort or fail to explore every avenue for its relief. But realistically, the physician is likely to have a greater effect on the parents than on the child.

Consequently, parents' stories about their pediatricians tend to fall into three categories: those who felt their pediatricians were not much help because they were not very concerned about colic as a health problem for the child or as a stress problem for the family; those whose pediatricians gave them specific help and advice . . . which didn't work; and those whose pediatricians gave them specific medical and counseling support that the parents felt made it easier for them to endure the colic.

In the category of remedies that didn't work, one woman said, "Our doctor gave us paregoric once, but nothing happened to the colic." In these cases we must acknowledge that the lack of an effect may not be due to the doctor or the suggested remedy, but to the nature of each particular child's colic. Since there may be several dozen medications, diet manipulations, and home therapies, and since some babies respond to some remedies and some to others, and most respond to none at all . . . obviously doctors have many more chances to miss than they do to hit.

One mother reported that her pediatrician "told us to calm down. He gave us some medicine for the baby, which didn't help. And because I was nursing, he told me to stop using dairy products, but there was no improvement then, either."

A mother at a New England air force base said, "Our doctor gave us some medication that we tried one night and it knocked him out completely; it really scared us. We tried a formula as a supplement to my nursing, but that didn't work. Then we tried feeding the baby peppermint spirits in water to bring up his gas, but that didn't have an effect, either."

Whether the remedies worked or not, these mothers were getting specific "things to do"—which has a therapeutic effect for the parents as well as a ghost of a chance of working for the child. But other women felt their pediatricians were uninterested:

One woman said, "Our doctor told us, 'He'll grow out of it.' " Another: "He told us, 'Ah, don't worry about it.' " (To her credit, she took his advice: "We assumed it would end," she said. And the colic, though it was bad while it lasted, went away at two and a half months.) And another mother: "Our pediatrician told us, 'Put him in his room and shut the door.' "

Although parents may feel offended by such abruptness, there are reasons for a physician's seeming lack of interest in colic. He or she knows the condition is neither dangerous nor prolonged, and that it will resolve by itself. And many doctors are overworked: When they are confronted with a case they know is not serious, they simply blurt out some advice, wash their hands, and move on to the next one. Their assessment and their advice are usually accurate—it's their manner and their choice of words that can make parents feel they have gotten short shrift. Counseling and support of worried parents takes *time* . . . just listening patiently is a major part of the therapy for frantic parents. But overextended physicians in large practices tend not to have that kind of time, and so are less able to support parents effectively.

Parents are grateful to physicians for detailed information, for a sympathetic hearing, and for advice that works. Unfortunately, in dealing with infant colic pediatricians have little control over what works, and consequently their advice will often be very general . . . and sometimes just plain lucky.

- "Our doctor told us to feed the baby very slowly, and in small amounts, about every two hours," a North Carolina mother recalled. "And we tried the different formulas. The baby ate pretty normally."
- A pediatrician in a suburb of Boston told one woman, "Be patient," and tried phenobarbital and formula changes for her infant's colic. "He also told us to wrap the baby up tightly in a soft, thin blanket, and that did work a little," she remembered.
- Another mother's pediatrician advised her to keep her colicky son on breast milk and soy milk, and to feed him a mild mixture of sugar water in a bottle. "It worked pretty well," she said.
- A woman whose daughter's colic lasted five months said, "We had been using a warm pad on the baby's belly without much change. But all along the doctor was reassuring me and complimenting me and that boosted me a lot."

The same remedy can seem like a lifesaver to some parents and a waste of time to others. One mother deeply appreciated her pediatrician's prescription of Sedadrops, the intestinal antispasmodic, while it was still being used for colic. She was a professional nurse who acknowledged "you use great care" with medications for infants, but she thought it helped. A woman whose children's colic lasted somewhat longer reported that her use of Sedadrops "never did that much good," even before its use for colic was discontinued.

The Pennsylvania father described nearly ideal pediatric support:

> *When our daughter first started shrieking and writhing, we took her to a pediatrician who said it was colic, that there was nothing he could do for it, and that we'd just have to "bite the bullet." Of course he was right, but we were so angry at what we thought was his uncaring attitude that we found another pediatrician, a guy who had just opened a new clinic and didn't have many patients yet. The paint still smelled fresh in the halls.*
>
> *Whenever we were in trouble with colic, he invited us to call him up, day or night, and describe our daughter's behavior: the screaming and twisting and so on. He'd say, Well, what are you doing for it? I'd tell him, for instance, My wife's got her in the living room and they're running the vacuum cleaner. The doctor would say, Is it working? Then we'd switch—my wife would get on the telephone and I'd go outside and walk the baby up and down the huge staircase that ran up the hill beside our house. What's happening? the doctor would ask. My wife would tell him, They're outside walking up and down the staircase.*
>
> *A few minutes later when my legs got tired and the baby was still screaming, we'd switch again, and I'd take the telephone. The doctor would say, Didn't work, huh? Where are they now? I'd tell him, They're down in the basement with the baby on top of the washer, doing a load*

> *of clothes. How's it going? he'd ask. I'd go to the door at the top of the basement stairs, listen for a moment, then go back to the telephone. She's still screaming, I'd tell him.*
>
> *This went on several times a week for months, like a vaudeville routine, until the colic tapered off by itself.*

The interviews for this book revealed a few physicians who were abrupt or unsympathetic with parents; perhaps such attitudes stemmed from their knowledge that colic will resolve itself, in time. But overwhelmingly, the pediatricians interviewed and those described by parents were supportive, encouraging, patient, and understanding of parents' anxiety and fatigue.

A number of physicians still feel that colic has a psychosomatic origin, either in the infant itself or in the parents, and that therefore the most effective approach is the "psychological" treatment, "talking through" the problem very patiently with the parents. Although this view of the origin of infant colic is not supported by recent research evidence, no parent who finds such a pediatrician will ever feel slighted in terms of the time and attention the doctor gives to the family.

The idea of talking to others—to seek advice, sympathy, or simply to express your fears about your baby's colic—is a vitally important therapy for the parent. Above all else, *do not* let your situation at home isolate you. Talk to your family and friends. Use the telephone. Call acquaintances at your church or synagogue, your Lamaze class, the La Leche League. Call your pediatrician and describe the day's routine.

Take a break when you can—ask a friend or neighbor to come in for half an hour while you nap or go for a walk.

After hearing your tales of woe, your friends will want to feel they can help you in some overt way.

But when friends and family have gone home and the doctor has hung up the telephone, you often find yourself back at square one. The evening stretches ahead and the colicky child is revving up. What are you going to do?

Tricks and Gimmicks

"I mean, we tried *every*thing. And *none* of it worked!"

The colic strategies that parents try at home seem after all to fall into two categories: those that help and those that don't. And some unfortunate parents, no matter what they do, fail to find a gimmick that will provide the baby and themselves with relief.

"We tried wrapping her up real tight," a mother said. "It made no difference. Rocking her made no difference. Warmth had no effect."

But parents who can't find the key—if there is one—to providing temporary relief must remember to give each therapy a fair chance to work and not to jump frantically from one trick to another, day by day. In fact, two or three out of the thirty-one infants sampled apparently responded very badly to *any* stimulation, and parents must be alert to the possibility that in some cases the best therapy is the least therapy, and a quiet, dim room with the gentlest handling may soothe the baby most.

And some parents make a deliberate decision not to drive themselves crazy trying to find a solution that may not exist. "With our first colicky daughter I tried so much that *didn't* work, that with our second colicky daughter I did very little but wait it out." This decision fits the pediatric advice, "There is nothing wrong with doing nothing."

Although many colicky infants seem to respond to the same three sensations—the motion of a baby swing, the security of tight infant carriers, and the warmth of baths or heating pads—there are always mavericks who respond only to some special trick that parents may stumble upon by trial and error or random luck.

"God's gift to parents is a pacifier with Karo syrup on it," one mother said. She also said that her colicky son was soothed by rocking, but not forward-and-back rocking. "He liked rocking from side to side, and I remember sitting there in the dark rocking from left to right at three o'clock in the morning."

Because of the nature of infant colic, the success of home remedies is highly relative. Even a gimmick that works only some of the time—and then only temporarily—can be judged a real winner.

"I sang a lot," one mother reported, "and I put him in a front pack so he'd doze off as I walked around. He might sleep four hours a day, but only in fifteen-minute catnaps."

Clearly one of the most popular items for calming colicky babies was the cloth infant carrier worn on the adult's chest. "I put her in the infant carrier because she'd scream too hard to hold a pacifier," a mother related. "Then I'd dance in the living room until she quieted down enough to take the pacifier."

The same mother said, "She was always a nonsleeper. We'd put quilts underneath her and she seemed to sleep easier. Swaddling or a very tight infant carrier often helped. The body contact seemed to be important."

Other parents agreed: "The front pack was a lifesaver," one woman reported. "At least she'd go to sleep in it." And she found the crank-up swing useful: "The motion seemed to help. Also, riding in the car was calming." Like other parents, she too learned to put the colicky baby in an infant seat on top of the washing machine while she was doing a load of laundry. The parents of colicky children may find their utilities budget takes a beating until the colic ends, but most will claim it's a small price to pay if it purchases a calmer infant.

"The cloth carrier? He hated it!" another mother said, proving there is no such thing as a universal colic remedy. "But the baby swing, that did help, from about two weeks on." She also recalled, "Other than the baby swing, he was too sensitive to stimulation. He didn't adjust to going places and being around people."

Other mothers found the baby swing helpful, too, even if it could not be called an unlimited success: "It helped him fall asleep for a half-hour at a time," one woman said, "so it did give me a break."

"The automatic swing helped as he got to two or three months," another recalled. "Also a bath in warm water helped, and wrapping him up tightly."

"The wind-up swing would work if she wasn't already crying too hard," an Indiana mother said. "Even at three days old, we would prop her up in it with pillows. We tried swaddling, but it didn't really help. Driving around in the car often calmed her down."

"A baby swing helped get us through supper," a Massachusetts woman reported; "but it didn't always work."

Even the commonest therapies do not work with all children. "We walked her up and down, we rode her in the car, we sat her near the washing machine," one parent said. "None of it worked. But if my husband sat in the rocking chair with his shirt open and held her against his chest, nine times out of ten she'd go to sleep."

Another woman recalls: "All I could do was walk and walk, talking to her and bouncing her around."

And another: "Any kind of stimulation was *terrible*. But the warm water bottle on her abdomen helped, and walking with my hand pressed against her belly worked."

A number of parents mentioned that the warmth of a bath or a heating pad was the most soothing thing they could do for their colicky children. "Neither of my kids would touch a pacifier," one woman told us, "but we'd put our colicky son in the bathtub every night; the warm water relaxed him and he'd pass some gas. This would be at nine or ten o'clock, for about half an hour. Then I could nurse him and put him to bed."

Another mother agreed: "We'd put a warm water bottle on his belly, then wrap him tight in a blanket, and it usually gave him some relief." Naturally parents must be very careful that warm pads aren't too warm, and that tight swaddling doesn't cut off blood circulation in the child's arms and legs.

"A warm pad would give us five to thirty minutes of relief," one parent recalled, "and a warm bath at eight P.M. really worked. He hushed at bath time."

"I had to hold a pacifier in his mouth," another said, "but it helped. He really liked a warm bath and tight blankets."

Sometimes, by watching the colicky baby carefully and experimenting gently, parents can invent effective therapies. Several parents have reported they got good results by kneading or massaging their babies' lower abdomens with their fingertips or palms. But one father went further: with his infant daughter on her back, he pushed her legs up so her knees pressed against her lower belly. His wife reported, "Most of the time she'd pass gas, but even if she didn't, it seemed to help." How did the father think of the idea? "I don't know," he said, "it just seemed like it would work." His wife recalled: "He was just sort of operating on instinct."

Nearly all parents of colicky infants have heard that feeding the baby a minuscule amount of brandy or liquor, mixed with sugar water or syrup, may help relax the child's intestines. Although we talked to several parents who had tried it, we failed to find a case where it had done any good.

A mother whose daughter's colic lasted five months reported, "I'd hold her real tight, I'd rock her hard, we'd walk outside, we'd go for a drive in the car . . . one night we were so frustrated we put a little vodka in her bottle . . . just a drop." Did it work? "Nope."

And a father recalled: "I think a pediatrician gave us that advice. We mixed a tiny amount of bourbon or brandy with some honey and warm water, and fed it like a syrup. It backfired. She was awake for hours, screaming and smelling like a Skid Row bum."

One of the experts in finding colic remedies was a mother of five children, the first four of whom were colicky:

"When our oldest girl was born I tried to nurse but I was really too young and too nervous. Like the other colicky kids she was worst from six to ten P.M., for about three months, then had afternoon fussiness, which lasted another three months. We used to massage her stomach to get rid of a lot of the gas, or use an enema to relax a tight sphincter muscle."

Her second colicky child seemed constantly constipated, and the mother used commercial suppositories. "She woke up at night a great deal. All my kids are different in all ways, and I learned you have to approach each child differently."

A third girl, born in Germany, was fed warm water in a bottle with peppermint flavoring. "It worked, helping her burp and relieving the gas. She'd burp once after nursing and half an hour later she'd have several *big* burps. I think it's important to be patient with the burping of a colicky child."

The mother reported that her only boy, the next born,

"woke up at night the longest." A warm water bottle after nursing "helped him burp ten times better," she said, "and helped thin out the milk."

The woman said that her family has a history of asthma related partly to an overproduction of mucous in the body. She shares the view of a number of athletes, physicians, nutritionists, and other parents that a diet heavy in milk and milk products generates excess mucous in the chest and nasal passages, and that colic or colicky behavior is an offshoot of the "thickening effect" of milk consumption. (A mother of two colicky boys agrees: "This is the first year I didn't require them to have milk with all three meals, and I think their health is the best it has ever been.")

A fifth child, a girl, was born at home in 1978: "I had no problems, ever, during labor. I had no bleeding at birth. The baby slept through the night from the absolute beginning. The child was at home, comfortable, no shots, no lights, sleeping in the same bed she was born into. . . ."

With her colicky children, the mother believed that "warm water, given after feedings, was the key" to breaking up the mucous and the undigested milk. "And you have to burp them very carefully over half an hour or more." She said, "None of my kids ever spit up. They were all big kids at birth, and they wanted to suck but it didn't seem to satisfy them. They ate a lot, and then they'd cry again."

The mother contends that parents can cope best with several children by involving the older ones in the care of the younger ones and the management of the house. "It's not always easy," she said. "I had three children under three years of age when I had gall bladder surgery, then moved to a new town. But you let the older kids help—teach them how to be useful and keep them interested. They can make jams and jellies, they can wash food and use the clothes washer, they can help potty-train the babies."

She pointed out one other skill the mothers of several young children learn: "Particularly if you have to carry a colicky baby around a lot, you learn to use your feet . . . to pick things up, close cabinet doors, and move furniture."

All these tactics have been designed to provide relief to the colicky child, and none can be guaranteed. But remember you can get relief by *getting away from the baby.*

If family finances permit it, signing up for a weekly activity even in advance of the baby's birth is a way of making a commitment to getting out, and to make getting out part of a weekly routine.

"We took disco lessons to get out, and then I went back to work when the baby was seven weeks old," one mother said. And another said, "I signed up for a night course and got out of the house."

"I was back at work in a month," one woman reported, "so I got out, all right." The problem was, she said, her job took a lot of energy, the colicky baby took the rest, and she was perpetually exhausted until her daughter's colic ended at four months.

The mother whose baby cried "all night long" for five months said, "I couldn't leave him with anybody. I had gone back to work, but I quit again and stayed home for a while, then went back to work when he was six months old."

There is no formula for getting away from a colicky infant, and even parents who know that it is important find it difficult to do: it's hard to find the energy to get out, hard to "impose" the screaming infant on a friend or baby-sitter, hard to leave a baby who seems so desperately unhappy. But leaving your colicky baby with a baby-sitter may be more unnerving for you than for the sitter.

Three things will help put your mind at ease. First, leave explicit instructions with the baby-sitter to let the child cry; once the baby's bottom is dry and its belly is full, putting it down in its crib to cry will do no damage to anyone. Second, for your reassurance and the sitter's, leave a telephone number where you can be reached while you are out. Third, if you don't have a twenty-eight-year-old friend willing to baby-sit, two fourteen-year-olds will do. One young teenager might get a little frazzled by a colicky child's incessant screaming, but two teenagers can reinforce each other; the bit of extra money you must spend will be well worth it in terms of your peace of mind.

Parents must learn the value of getting out to rediscover their adult lives and interests, or the pleasure of rediscovering their other children by taking them to a playground or pool. As the pediatricians say, you can't be effective with a colicky child when you are fatigued and overstressed. So sometimes the best thing you can do for the infant is to take yourself away for a few hours, in order to increase your effectiveness when you return.

At their pediatrician's suggestion, virtually every parent interviewed had been through the "process of elimination" suggested by Lawrence Breslow's research: ruling out first hunger and feeding technique as possible causes of the colic, then carbohydrates and butterfats, then allergies, and so on. In truth, this is a routine that most pediatricians contend you must go through "just in case . . ." But a true resolution of colic by this method is quite rare.

Remember that you're looking for the tactics that will work with your particular baby. Hopefully, you can quickly find some remedies that will ease the colicky behavior. But if you expect the first gimmick to work—or the tenth—the odds are you'll be disappointed.

Each child may respond to a different remedy: one to a warm water bottle after feedings, one to a belly massage and patient burping, another to measures to relieve gas or constipation. Since the colic itself may be idiosyncratic from child to child, it would seem that the parents who are adaptable and persistent stand the best chance of finding an effective therapy.

When you try these devices, don't run through the whole list in two days; give each trick a fair chance to work, over at least five or six days. And there may be combinations that will soothe or lull your baby—perhaps an infant swing set out in the sunshine will be more effective than rocking the child in a dim room.

You can add your own inventions to this list of other parents' "old favorites":

- keeping the baby's room dim and quiet, and the child free of stimulation
- using a pacifier with Karo syrup on it
- swaddling or wrapping the baby with a thin blanket
- rocking the baby, forward and back or side to side
- holding the baby tightly, for close personal contact
- putting a warm water bottle or heating pad on the infant's belly
- sitting the baby up, virtually all the time, to aid the movement of food and the passage of gas
- the "front-pack" cloth baby carrier
- the automatic, wind-up baby swing

- sitting the baby on the washing machine while you do the laundry
- driving in the car, to lull the child into drowsiness
- massaging the baby's belly with your fingertips, or pressing the infant's knees upward against its stomach, or pressing the child's lower belly with your fingers as you walk or rock
- giving the baby a warm water bottle after its regular feeding
- patient burping
- diet alterations, both for the infant and the nursing mother
- getting away from the child as often as you can arrange it

The tricks and gimmicks can be counted on to work—sometimes. But all bets are off in the special cases where infant colic is complicated by circumstances in the home environment, the family, or the child itself.

Special Cases

In some colic situations the parents simply cannot get away—for example, the parents of premature colicky twins—and in other cases no amount of pediatric support and encouragement can change basic family circumstances such as extreme poverty or overcrowding at home.

Dr. David Reynolds, for example, practiced in pediatric clinics in Portsmouth, Virginia, near the huge Norfolk Naval Base. He noted that because of the special nature of military reservations, pediatric office visits followed a pattern: the father was not there, the mother's family was hundreds or thousands of miles away, and the family's financial situation was marginal. "That's a combination of stresses that can lead to problems in any case," said Reynolds, "with or without colic."

Dr. Tom Murphy, a pediatrician who practiced at a U.S. air base on the island of Okinawa in the South Pacific, agreed that in such circumstances the physician must tailor his recommendations to what is *realistically* possible. "Sure, you could tell the mother to get out of the house and go bowling three times a week," he recalled, "but you had to consider, one, could she afford it; two, could she afford a babysitter; three, could she even *find* a babysitter?"

One of the barriers to consistent medical care, Murphy pointed out, is that families in the military—particularly young ones—move about so rapidly. "You'd open someone's medical record folder and see thirty-five visits to fifteen different physicians," he said. Family visits to many medical practices negate the planned, methodical approach that colic seems to respond to best.

But family circumstances need not be that dramatic in order to make infant colic far more difficult to cope with. One common source of extra tension and anxiety is the burden of moving a household while caring for a colicky infant. A husband's absence is another common circumstance that magnifies the difficulty of coping with a colicky child, and complicating health factors in the family constitute yet another source of anxiety.

In such stressful circumstances both the physicians and the parents interviewed for this book agreed that there is only one choice: use your pediatrician for support and counseling. Where a pediatric practice is not available for some reason, there are usually family practice physicians, licensed nurse practitioners or physicians' assistants, or the outpatient departments of hospitals or public health departments.

The Children Later: A Joy to Behold

Given the anxiety and concern that colicky infants cause their parents, how do mothers characterize these children as they get older?

"As an infant he couldn't stand to be held," an inner-city mother said. "I was afraid he would be aloof or hyperactive." Instead, as her once-colicky son turned two, she described a "warm and affectionate" child who was also "very intense, serious, alert, and active."

Discovering who our children are may be the most fascinating aspect of parenthood. There was usually a slight note of surprise and wonderment in parents' voices as they searched for words to describe their former colic cases. "He's precocious, verbal, and intense . . . not athletic . . . but pretty intellectual," a mother said of her seven-year-old.

Three words kept cropping up in the conversations about the children as they grew and developed: outgoing, active, and intense. Perhaps those terms characterize most American kids in their preschool and school years. But some parents were clearly describing differences between their colicky and non-colicky children: "She's a skinny kid, very outgoing, and more active than our other child," one mother said of her four-and-a-half-year-old, who was the younger of her two.

Some of the children retained behavior patterns that are often a part of colic—particularly sleeplessness. "She was not a good sleeper as an infant, and she still isn't," one mother said of her three-year-old. "She'll get up at eight and go to bed at nine P.M., without a nap. If she does nap, I'll put her to bed at nine and turn out the light, and ninety minutes later you'll hear her in there talking and singing and playing, until she drifts off."

Another mother similarly described her two colicky children when the older was eight and a half years and the younger was eight and a half months: "The older one is large, shy but active, not 'hyper,' but not a real sleeper, either. The younger one is also large, precocious physically, active, and not a sleeper . . . quite wakeful."

A second characteristic that seemed to carry over from the children's colicky days was a big appetite: "He's a good eater," said one mother of her son at age ten. "He's *very* active and outgoing, and loves to run." Another woman said her once-colicky daughter "will eat anything" at eighteen months. She said the girl was "above average in height and weight; she's very happy and active."

Even the children who had been highly allergic to milk, milk products, and eggs as infants were described by their mothers as "normal, fast-growing, active and outgoing," although some retained a slight milk intolerance into their school years.

Several parents described rough-and-tumble kids, boys and girls. The woman who reported that she had to quit work again after going back, because she couldn't leave her colicky son with anyone, described him at fifteen months as a child who "eats anything and sleeps well," had "great" health, and was "good, playful, loves running . . . he walked at eight and a half months . . ."

A three-year-old boy who was colicky for six months was described by his mother as "big, very active and very healthy," and "outgoing, overambitious and accident prone." An eight-year-old girl was described by her father: "She's very energetic physically—loves roller skating and swimming. She's also an unusually talented artist, and has a very inquiring mind in her reading and the way she looks at nature. But headstrong . . . I've never seen a kid as opinionated, willful, and argumentative."

Of course all of these descriptions would fit non-colicky children as well, and obviously no "predictive" value can be attached to them. But because we are investigating children who were a huge pain in the neck to their parents as infants, it's fun and interesting to see how they "turn out" as they grow older.

The mother of a two-and-a-half-year-old said that her daughter "goes to a day-care center, loves books, talks up a storm, and was a very early walker." Another described two once-colicky boys: "Both are gregarious and outgoing, and creative. The first is ten years old, very active and precocious, a goer. The second is ten months old, quieter and not as active, and seems to concentrate longer."

As in everything else about colic, just as we think patterns are beginning to emerge—kids who are intense and active—we find another subset of once-colicky children who are also active, but are described by their parents as easy-going and good-natured.

The mother of a colicky girl said that at age two she was "very active and very affectionate"; another mother of two colicky children described them, when one was twenty years old and the other was eighteen months, as "good eaters but not as active . . . both are so sweet and gentle."

A fourteen-month-old girl who "eats well and grows well" was described by her mother as "not shy . . . the best-natured baby I've ever seen."

The overwhelming picture that emerges of these children is that they are entirely normal and healthy and active kids. Like all children, they can still worry and frustrate their parents ("accident prone," "argumentative"), but also like all children, their activity and creativity is a joy to their mothers and fathers.

A Final Word

Parents' experiences indicate that it's helpful to believe —almost as a matter of faith—that *something* will help relieve colic if you persist steadfastly in the search. That belief in itself helps many parents get through . . . and it's not just a matter of inspiration. We know that no colic remedy works with all children, but we also know that some tactics do work with some children. The relief of colic is not just a lottery—you do what you sensibly can, to help your baby and help yourself.

Parents of colicky children discover that they do have resources, and that the problem is not in their competence or their love for the child. As one mother explained, such confidence is a major source of energy in enduring infant colic. Another said, "You have to keep your perspective and your sense of humor."

If you don't feel very confident or humorous—and that's understandable—look systematically for the resources that do exist. Above all, don't retreat into a cycle of isolation and fatigue, confusion and despair. Talk to people. Call your pediatrician and tell him or her what you are thinking and feeling. Call your family and neighbors, and tell them what you need. Call your clergyman or a local parents' group, and state your worst fears out loud.

The single best aspect of infant colic is that the condition has a happy ending: the kid is going to outgrow it.

The screaming will end, and parents and child will discover the peace, love, and comfort they have wanted from each other.

What is infant colic? Two characteristics stand out. First: it's an absolute terror while it lasts. Second: it's going to go away, and years from now you'll chuckle when you tell friends how you got through it. That's only fair. It's the parents' reward for surviving the colic.

Bibliography

Listed below are the better and more recent articles related to infant colic or colic symptoms. The best are noted with an asterisk.

Aldrich, C. A., Sung, C., and Knop, C. "The Crying of Newly Born Babies." *Journal of Pediatrics* 27 (1945): 428–35.

* Brackett, A. S. "The Alleviation of Pylorospasm and Colic in Infants by Reducing the Volume of the Food Intake per Feeding." *Yale Journal of Biology and Medicine* 19 (1946): 155–69.

* ———. "Enteric Colic." *Yale Journal of Biology and Medicine* 20 (1948): 553–66.

Brazelton, T. B. "Crying in Infancy." *Pediatrics* 29 (1962): 579–88.

Breslow, Lawrence. "A Clinical Approach to Infantile Colic." *Journal of Pediatrics* 57 (1957): 196–206.

Buisseret, P. D. "Common Manifestations of Cow's Milk Allergy in Children." *The Lancet* 1 (1978): 304–05.

Carey, W. B. "Maternal Anxiety and Infantile Colic." *Clinical Pediatrics* 7 (1969): 590–95.

* Clark, R. L., Ganis, F. M., and Bradford, W. L. "A Study of the Possible Relationship of Progesterone to Colic." *Pediatrics* 31 (1963): 65–71.

Cleary, D. M. "When Your Baby Has Colic." *Today's Health*, February 1962, p. 54.

Committee on Nutrition, American Academy of Pediatrics. "The

Practical Significance of Lactose Intolerance in Children." *Pediatrics* 62 (1978): 240–45.

Du, J. N. H. "Colic as the Sole Symptom of Urinary Tract Infection in Infants." *Canadian Medical Association Journal* 115 (1976): 334–37.

Dworkin, P. H., Shonkoff, J. P., Leviton, A., and Levine, M. D. "Training in Developmental Pediatrics." *American Journal of Diseases of Children* 133 (1979): 709–12.

Escalona, S. K. "Feeding Disturbances in Very Young Children." *American Journal of Orthopsychiatry* 15 (1945): 76–80.

Farran, Christopher. "What Mothers Say About Colic." *Baby Talk*, March 1981, p. 28.

———, and Farran, Dale. "The Screaming Baby Blues." *Parents*, July 1981, p. 56.

Glaser, J. "Colic in Infants: Excerpts from a Panel Discussion." *Pediatrics* 18 (1956): 828–40.

Gordon, D. A. "The Hypertonic Child." *Archives of Pediatrics* 65 (1948): 70–83.

Harris, M. J., Petts, V., and Penny, R. "Cow's Milk Allergy as a Cause of Infantile Colic." *Australian Paediatric Journal* 13 (1977): 276–81.

Holmes, C. A. "Infantile Colic: A Practitioner's Interpretation." *Clinical Pediatrics* 8 (1969): 566–69.

* Illingworth, R. S. "Three Months' Colic." *Archives of Diseases in Childhood* 29 (1954): 165–74.

———. "Three Months' Colic: Treatment by Methylscopolamine Nitrate." *Acta Paediatrica* 44 (1955): 203–08.

———, and Leeds, M. D. "Evening Colic in Infants: A Double-Blind Trial of Dicyclomine Hydrochloride." *The Lancet* 2 (1959): 1119–20.

Jakobsson, I., and Lindberg, T. "Cow's Milk as a Cause of Infantile Colic in Breast-Fed Infants." *The Lancet* 2 (1978): 437–39.

Jorup, Sigvard. "Colonic Hyperperistalsis in Neurolabile Infants." *Acta Paediatrica* 41, suppl. 85 (1952): 596–99.

Keiter, W. E. "Colic (Gastro-Enterospasm)." *Virginia Medical Monthly* 65 (1938): 479–83.

Levin, Harris. "Infantile Colic in Institutions." *American Journal of Diseases of Children* 79 (1950): 666–72.

* Levine, Milton I., and Bell, Anita I. "The Treatment of 'Colic' in Infancy by Use of the Pacifier." *Journal of Pediatrics* 37 (1950): 750–55.

Liebman, W. M. "Infantile Colic: Association with Lactose and Milk Intolerance." *Journal of the American Medical Association* 245 (1981): 732–33.

———. "Recurrent Abdominal Pain in Children: Lactose and Sucrose Intolerance." *Pediatrics* 64 (1979): 43–45.

Lipton, E. L., Steinschneider, A., and Richmond, J. B. "Autonomic Function in the Neonate." *Psychosomatic Medicine* 22 (1960): 57–65.

* ———, and Steinschneider, A. "Swaddling: A Child Care Practice." *Pediatrics* suppl. (March 1965), 521–67.

Martin, F. J. "The Colicky Baby." *Annals of Allergy* 12 (1954): 700–03.

Meyer, J. E., and Thaler, M. M. "Colic in Low Birth Weight Infants." *American Journal of Diseases of Children* 122 (1971): 25–27.

Neff, F. C. "The Pharmacopeia and the Physician: The Treatment of Colic in Infants." *Journal of the American Medical Association* 114 (1940): 1745–48.

* O'Donovan, J. C., and Bradstock, A. S. "The Failure of Conventional Drug Therapy in the Management of Infantile Colic." *American Journal of Diseases of Children* 133 (1979): 999–1001.

* Paradise, J. L. "Maternal and Other Factors in the Etiology of Infantile Colic." *Journal of the American Medical Association* 197 (1966): 123–31.

Pierce, P. P. "Delayed Onset of Three Months' Colic in Premature Infants." *American Journal of Diseases of Children* 75 (1948): 190–92.

Roby, C. C., Ober, W. B., and Drorbaugh, J. E. "Pregnanediol Excretion in the Urine of Newborn Male Infants." *Pediatrics* 17 (1956): 877–81.

Rosamond, E. "Breast Fed Babies Who Cry at Night." *Southern Medical Journal* 14 (1921): 768–74.

Rowell, P. A. "Infantile Colic: Reviewing the Situation." *Pediatric Nursing* 4 (1978): 20–21.

Shannon, W. R. "Colic in Breast-Fed Infants as a Result of Sensitization to Foods in the Mother's Dietary." *Archives of Pediatrics* 38 (1921): 756–61.

Shaver, Benjamin A. "Maternal Personality and Early Adaptation to Infantile Colic." In *Psychological Aspects of a First Pregnancy and Early Postnatal Adapatation,* edited by P. M.

Shereshefsky and L. J. Yarrow. New York: Raven Press, 1974. Pages 209–15.

Snow, William. "The Postural Treatment of Infant Colic." *American Journal of Roentgenology* 38 (1937): 779–80.

Speer, Frederic. "Colic and Allergy: A Ten-Year Study." *Archives of Pediatrics* 75 (1958): 271–78.

Spock, Benjamin. "Etiological Factors in Hypertrophic Pyloric Stenosis and Infantile Colic." *Psychosomatic Medicine* 6 (1944): 162–65.

* Stendler, C. B. "Psychologic Aspects of Pediatrics: Sixty Years of Child Training Practices." *Journal of Pediatrics* 36 (1950): 122–34.

Stewart, A. H., Weiland, I. H., Leider, A. R., Mangham, C. A., Holmes, T. H., and Ripley, H. S. "Excessive Infant Crying (Colic) in Relation to Parent Behavior." *American Journal of Psychiatry* 110 (1954): 687–94.

Taylor, W. C. "A Study of Infantile Colic." *Canadian Medical Association Journal* 76 (1957): 458–61.

Townley, R. R. W. "Colic and Cow's Milk Allergy." *Australian Paediatric Journal* 13 (1977): 259–60.

Wessel, Morris A., Cobb, J. C., Jackson, E. B., Harris, G. S., and Detwiler, A. C. "Paroxysmal Fussing in Infancy, Sometimes Called 'Colic.'" *Pediatrics* 14 (1954): 421–34.

White, P. J. "The Classification and Treatment of Infantile Colic or Gastro-Enterospasm." *Medical Clinics of North America* 20 (1936): 511–25.

———. "Management of Infantile Colic." *American Journal of Diseases of Children* 133 (1979): 995–96.

———. "The Relation Between Colic and Eczema in Early Infancy." *American Journal of Diseases of Children* 38 (1929): 935–42.

Index